Recent Advances in

Surgery
35

)162.
fax 01
E-m

5

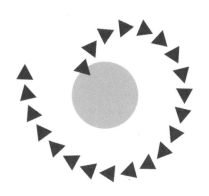

Recent Advances in

Surgery
35

Edited by

Colin D Johnson MChir FRCS
Reader in Surgery and Honorary Consultant Surgeon
University Surgical Unit
University Hospital Southampton
Southampton, UK

Irving Taylor MD ChM FRCS FMedSci FHEA
Professor of Surgery and Vice Dean
UCL Medical School
University College London
London, UK

JAYPEE BROTHERS MEDICAL PUBLISHERS (P) LTD

New Delhi • London • Philadelphia • Panama

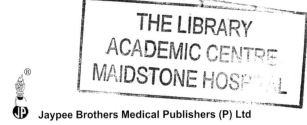

Jaypee Brothers Medical Publishers (P) Ltd

Headquarters

Jaypee Brothers Medical Publishers (P) Ltd
4838/24, Ansari Road, Daryaganj
New Delhi 110 002, India
Phone: +91-11-43574357
Fax: +91-11-43574314
Email: jaypee@jaypeebrothers.com

Overseas Offices

J.P. Medical Ltd
83, Victoria Street, London
SW1H 0HW (UK)
Phone: +44-2031708910
Fax: +02-03-0086180
Email: info@jpmedpub.com

Jaypee Brothers Medical Publishers Ltd
The Bourse
111 South Independence Mall East
Suite 835, Philadelphia, PA 19106, USA
Phone: + 267-519-9789
Email: joe.rusko@jaypeebrothers.com

Jaypee Brothers Medical Publishers (P) Ltd
Shorakhute, Kathmandu, Nepal
Phone: +00977-9841528578
Email: jaypee.nepal@gmail.com

Jaypee-Highlights Medical Publishers Inc.
City of Knowledge, Bld. 237, Clayton
Panama City, Panama
Phone: +507-301-0496
Fax: +507-301-0499
Email: cservice@jphmedical.com

Jaypee Brothers Medical Publishers (P) Ltd
17/1-B Babar Road, Block-B, Shaymali
Mohammadpur, Dhaka-1207
Bangladesh
Mobile: +08801912003485
Email: jaypeedhaka@gmail.com

Website: www.jaypeebrothers.com
Website: www.jaypeedigital.com

Inquiries for bulk sales may be solicited at: jaypee@jaypeebrothers.com

This book has been published in good faith that the contents provided by the contributors contained herein are original, and is intended for educational purposes only. While every effort is made to ensure accuracy of information, the publisher and the editors specifically disclaim any damage, liability, or loss incurred, directly or indirectly, from the use or application of any of the contents of this work. If not specifically stated, all figures and tables are courtesy of the editors. Where appropriate, the readers should consult with a specialist or contact the manufacturer of the drug or device.

Recent Advances in Surgery 35

First Edition: **2013**

ISBN: 978-93-5090-376-6

Printed at: Ajanta Offset & Packagings Ltd., New Delhi

Contributors

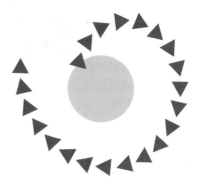

Anushka Chaudhry MBBS FRCS (Gen Surg)
Specialist Registrar in General Surgery
Division of Head and Neck Surgery
University Hospitals of Bristol NHS Foundation Trust
Bristol, Avon, UK

Avi Agrawal MBBS MSc FRCS (Ed) FRCS (Gen Surg)
Portsmouth Breast Care Centre
Queen Alexandra Hospital
Portsmouth, UK

Bateman AR MBBS MRCP FRCR PhD
Somers Cancer Research Building
University of Southampton Cancer Sciences Division
Southampton University Hospitals NHS Trust
Southampton, UK

CP Shearman BSc FRCS MS
Professor
Department of Vascular Surgery
University Hospital of Southampton NHS Foundation Trust
Southampton, UK

Christina Summerhayes MBBS BSc FRCS
Portsmouth Breast Care Centre
Queen Alexandra Hospital
Portsmouth, UK

D Bray FRCS (ORL-HNS)
Priory Barn
Hildenborough, Kent, UK

Declan FJ Dunne MBChB
Research Fellow
Aintree University Hospital
Longmoor Lane
Liverpool, UK

Graeme J Poston MSc MBChB FRCS
Consultant Liver Surgeon
Aintree University Hospital
Longmoor Lane
Liverpool, UK

Hamish Noble MS FRCS
Post CCT Fellow in Bariatric Surgery
Musgrove Park Hospital
Taunton, Somerset, UK

Iain Anderson BSc MD FRCS
Consultant Surgeon
Salford Royal Hospital
Stott Lane, Salford, UK

Jurgen J Mulsow MD FRCSI
Lecturer in Surgery
University College Dublin
Belfield, Dublin, Ireland
Consultant Surgeon
Mater Misericordiae University Hospital
Dublin 7, Ireland

Jyoti Shah BSc (Hons) MD MS DHMSA FRCS (Urol)
Consultant Urologist
Queen's Hospital
Staffordshire, UK

K Mylankal MD FRCS
Consultant Vascular Surgeon
Department of Vascular Surgery
University Hospital of Southampton NHS Foundation Trust
Southampton, UK

Keith Gardiner MD MCh FRCS
Consultant General, Colorectal and Intestinal Failure Surgeon
Colorectal and Intestinal Failure Unit
Royal Victoria Hospital
Belfast, UK

Kevin McElvanna MB MRCSI
Specialty Registrar
Colorectal and Intestinal Failure Unit
Royal Victoria Hospital
Belfast, UK

Malcolm West MD MRCS (Ed)
Clinical Research Fellow and Specialist Surgical Registrar
Aintree University Hospitals NHS Foundation Trust
Liverpool, UK

Michael PW Grocott BSc MBBS MD FRCA FRCP FFICM
Professor of Anaesthesia and Intensive Care
University Hospital Southampton NHS Foundation Trust
Southampton, UK

Mirnezami AH BSc BM PhD FRCS
Senior Lecturer and Consultant Colorectal Surgeon
Somers Cancer Research Building
University of Southampton Cancer Sciences Division
Southampton University Hospitals NHS Trust
Southampton, UK

Mirnezami R BSc MBBS MRCS
Section of Biosurgery and Surgical Technology
Department of Surgery and Cancer
Imperial College London
St Mary's Hospital
London, UK

P Ronan O'Connell MD FRCSI FRCPSGlas
Professor of Surgery
School of Medicine and Medical Science
St Vincent's University Hospital
Elm Park, Dublin 4, Ireland

Rachel Oeppen MB ChB MRCP FRCR
Southampton Breast Unit
University Southampton
Level C, Princess Anne Hospital
Southampton, UK

Ramsey I Cutress MA BM BCh PhD FRCS (Ed)
Consultant Breast Surgeon
University Hospital Southampton NHS Foundation Trust
Southampton, UK

Richard Welbourn MD FRCS
Consultant in Upper Gastrointestinal and Bariatric Surgery
Musgrove Park Hospital
Taunton, Somerset, UK

Robert P Jones BSc MBChB
Research Fellow
Aintree University Hospital
Longmoor Lane
Liverpool, UK

Sandy Jack MSc PhD
Consultant Clinical Scientist
Aintree University Teaching Hospitals NHS Foundation Trust
Liverpool, UK

S Ramkumar MD MRCPI FRCP FRCR
Department of Clinical Oncology
University Hospital Southampton Foundation Trust
Southampton, UK

Siân Pugh BSc (Hons) BM (Hons) MRCS
Academic Clinical Fellow in Surgery
University Surgical Unit
Southampton General Hospital
Southampton, UK

VK Kapoor FRCS FACS FACG
Professor of Surgical Gastroenterology
Sanjay Gandhi Postgraduate Institute of Medical Sciences
Lucknow, India

William Wallace MD FRCS
Specialist Registrar
Colorectal and Intestinal Failure Unit
Royal Victoria Hospital
Belfast, UK

Zoë Ellen Winters DPhil (Oxon) FRCS (Edin) FCS (SA) MBBCh (Rand)
Consultant Senior Lecturer in Breast Surgery
Director of the Breast Reconstruction Patient Reported
and Clinical Outcomes Research Group
School of Clinical Sciences
University of Bristol and Division of Head and Neck Surgery
University Hospitals of Bristol NHS Foundation Trust
Bristol, Avon, UK

Preface

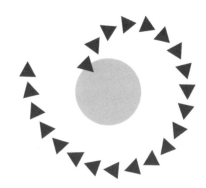

This latest volume of *Recent Advances in Surgery* follows a familiar pattern. We have invited contributions which address important and topical subjects in Surgery-in-General, and in the major subspecialities of General Surgery.

There is a strong section on Surgery-in-General, with reviews by experts in the fields of cardiopulmonary exercise testing in preoperative assessment, and perioperative care. In Gastrointestinal Surgery, we are including chapters on bariatric surgery, liver metastases, ischaemic bowel, anal cancer, intra-operative radiotherapy for rectal cancer and abdominal tuberculosis. Vascular Surgery is represented by consideration of the management of the diabetic foot, a growing problem worldwide. Reconstruction after surgery for breast cancer is an important area where the surgeon's skills remain indispensable.

As always, we conclude with a wide-ranging look through randomised clinical trials and meta-analyses published last year.

We believe that this volume maintains the high standards of the past, and we are confident that it will be valued by practicing surgeons and examination candidates in General Surgery.

Colin D Johnson
Irving Taylor

Contents

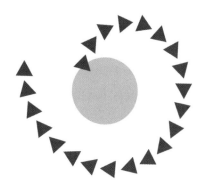

1

Perioperative Care

Jyoti Shah

INTRODUCTION

There were 6,954,241 surgical operations and procedures carried out in the UK in 2010-11.[1] Although the overall risk of death and major complications after surgery is low,[2] the majority of deaths (80%) occur in a small group of high-risk patients.[3]

Surgeons are under growing pressure to increase day case surgery and reduce inpatient hospital stays. The Modernisation Agency High Impact change No. 1 recognises that at least 80% of patients undergoing elective surgery could be treated as day cases and states that this should be the norm for elective surgery. Coupled with factors such as an ageing population, greater co-morbidities and complex surgical procedures, a multidisciplinary team approach is essential to achieve satisfactory results. There is good evidence that patient outcome after major noncardiac surgery can be considerably improved with effective perioperative care.[4] But what do we mean by perioperative care? The perioperative period incorporates the patient's entire surgical experience. It starts at the point a patient is listed and thus consented for an operation, and extends into their postoperative recovery. The best outcome can only be achieved with attention to detail at every stage of this journey.

> **Key Point**
>
> Perioperative care incorporates the patient's entire surgical journey and includes pre-, peri- and postoperative care.

PREOPERATIVE ASSESSMENT

The fundamental purpose of preoperative evaluation is to obtain information about the patient's medical history and background, formulate an assessment of their surgical risk and minimise cancellations on the day of surgery (Table 1.1). The preoperative visit may also relieve anxiety and answer any questions about the operation and the anaesthetic.[5] In a recent publication, 16% of UK hospitals had no preadmission anaesthetic assessment clinic and 17% had no surgical assessment clinic.[6]

TABLE 1.1: Benefits of effective preassessment

Ensure patients are fully informed about their proposed operation
Estimate the level of risk from an anaesthetic
Check consent
Identify co-existing illnesses and optimise them
Identify high-risk patients
Undertaken relevant investigations
Reduce patient's anxiety
Reduce cancellations on the day of surgery
Plan discharge

Many of these clinics are nurse-led and are essential for the assessment of a patient before elective surgery. They also provide an opportunity to ensure patients know and understand the procedure scheduled to be carried out, and the risks involved. A full discussion of the consenting process is beyond the scope of this chapter, but readers are reminded that good surgical practice incorporates the following principles:

1. Describes the procedure, usually in the outpatient setting
2. Discusses probability of risks and likely complications
3. Discusses associated risks such as those from an anaesthetic, need for intravenous fluids or catheters, etc.
4. Describes alternatives to the proposed operation and the likely prognosis if the patient declines surgery. Failure to provide sufficient information can result in a claim in negligence.[7]

> **Key Point**
>
> Preassessment clinics are essential to screen patients for fitness for an anaesthetic and surgery.

IDENTIFYING RISK

There are a number of ways of stratifying risk preoperatively in patients scheduled for surgery. Of these, the American Society of Anaesthesiologists (ASA) grading of physical status (PS) on a scale of 1 to 6 is the simplest and most widely used. It was originally introduced in 1941, and has since undergone modifications such that an additional suffix 'E' has been added for patients undergoing emergency surgery (Table 1.2).[8]

TABLE 1.2: American Society of Anaesthesiologists (ASA) physical status (PS) classification

ASA PS 1	Normal healthy patients
ASA PS 2	Patients with mild systemic disease
ASA PS 3	Patients with severe systemic disease
ASA PS 4	Patients with severe systemic disease that is a constant threat to life
ASA PS 5	Moribund patients not expected to survive without the operation
ASA PS 6	Patients declared brain-dead whose organs are being removed for donor purposes
E	Patients undergoing emergency surgery

The ASA grade is a subjective tool that provides an indication of relative risk of surgery to the patient. However, it does not actually quantify the risk as a patient undergoing excision of a skin lesion under local anaesthetic will have the same ASA grade for this as they would with major bowel surgery. Hence, the ASA grade cannot be used as the sole predictor of operative risk. It can also change from when the patient was seen in clinic to the actual time of surgery. Interestingly, it fails to take account of age, weight, malignancy or the results of any laboratory tests, and is based on history alone. It seems to omit risk for patients with moderate disease allowing for only mild and severe.

Although other more complex and time-consuming classifications exist, the ASA grade is relatively robust having stood the test of time, and is used commonly to communicate patient risk between doctors.

DETECTING DISEASE

Several investigators have demonstrated the costly overuse of routine investigations for healthy patients undergoing elective surgery. Almost 30 years ago, Kaplan and colleagues reviewed the laboratory screening results of 2,000 patients booked for elective surgery. They found that 60% of these tests were unnecessary and only 0.22% revealed abnormalities that might influence perioperative management.[9] Similarly, in a review of 2,570 patients with 5,003 preoperative screening test results, only four patients were believed to have a conceivable benefit from those tests.[10] Unnecessary preoperative investigations are associated with problems other than cost and waste. Doctors do not always check the results of requested investigations, and many requests are duplicated. In a study reviewing the results of 7,549 preoperative tests in 1,109 patients who had elective surgery, the authors demonstrated that 47% of these tests were duplicated and unnecessary.[11] Additionally, false positive results can lead to unnecessary, costly and potentially harmful treatments, further investigations and cancellation of operations.[12]

The National Institute of Healthcare and Clinical Excellence (NICE) recommends the following preoperative tests based on surgical severity (Table 1.3).[13]

- Full blood count: In patients aged over 60 years and surgical severity 2 or more, all patients with surgical severity 3 or more and severe renal disease
- Serum electrolytes: Serum creatinine is elevated in 0.2–2.4% of asymptomatic patients.[14] NICE recommends routine testing of creatinine in patients aged over 60 years and surgical severity 3 or more, all patients with surgical severity grade 4 and all patients with renal or cardiovascular disease
- Sickle cell test: All patients of African, Afro-Caribbean, Asian, Middle-Eastern or East-Mediterranean ancestry

- Pregnancy test: All women of child-bearing age (regardless of history)
- Electrocardiogram (ECG): In a large study of 23,036 patients undergoing 28,457 surgical procedures, the absolute difference in the incidence of cardiovascular death between those with and those without ECG abnormalities was only 0.5%, thereby questioning the benefit of its routine use.[15] NICE recommends its use in patients aged over 80 years, those over 60 years of age and surgical severity of 3 or more, and any patient with cardiovascular disease or severe renal disease
- Chest X-ray (CXR): In a meta-analysis of 21 studies that included review of 14,390 routine preoperative CXR films, 1.3% of films had unexpected abnormalities, causing modification of management in only 0.1%.[16] Routine use of CXR is recommended in patients undergoing cardiac or major abdominal surgery, or in patients with respiratory disease.

TABLE 1.3: Surgical severity[13]

Surgical severity	Examples of surgical procedures
Grade 1	Diagnostic procedures – endoscopy, laparoscopy, breast biopsy
Grade 2	Inguinal hernia repair, varicose veins, adenotonsillectomy, knee arthroscopy
Grade 3	Total abdominal hysterectomy, transurethral prostatectomy, lumbar discectomy, thyroidectomy
Grade 4	Total joint replacement, vascular reconstruction, colonic resection, radical neck dissection

Evidence, however, points to history and examination performed by trained staff as the most efficient way of detecting disease. In a general medical clinic, the correct diagnosis was established in 56% of patients after taking a good history. Physical examination increased this figure to 73% and routine laboratory investigations only helped to make the diagnosis in 5% of patients whilst significantly increasing cost.[17]

> **Key Point**
>
> Laboratory tests should not be repeated for elective surgery if the results were normal within 4 months, providing there has been no change to the patient's condition.

JEHOVAH'S WITNESSES

The absolute refusal of whole blood and major blood components is a core value of the 140,000 Jehovah's witnesses in the UK. They will usually identify themselves in the preoperative setting and clarify their own decision regarding blood products, often producing a detailed advance directive. A thorough discussion of the risks of surgery is essential when the patient is a competent adult, usually with local representatives from the Jehovah's Witness Hospital Liaison Committee. A specific Department of Health consent form must be completed and the acceptability of various fluids should be documented and respected. Whole blood, packed red cells, platelets, white blood cells, plasma and 'predonation' of blood for later autotransplantation is not acceptable, whereas fractions of blood products such as albumin, immunoglobulin, vaccines, clotting factors and prothrombin complex concentrates may be.[18] Various pre-, intra- and postoperative measures need to be considered to minimise the risk of bleeding.[18]

OBESITY

The prevalence of obesity worldwide is increasing and therefore surgeons are likely to see more obese patients presenting for surgery. Obesity is defined as body mass index (BMI) > 30 kg/m^2 (Table 1.4).

TABLE 1.4: Definition of obesity

Body mass index (BMI) (kg/m^2)	Description
< 25	Normal
25–30	Overweight
30–35	Obese
> 35	Morbidly obese
> 55	Supermorbidly obese

Patients with an elevated BMI have a high prevalence of co-morbid conditions (50% hypertension, 25% asthma, 50% arthritis, 30% diabetes), thereby increasing their operative morbidity. This group has an 'all cause of death' hazard ratio of upto 3.[19] Risk reduction begins with careful case selection for surgery, taking a detailed history focusing on evidence of snoring, daytime somnolence and sleep patterns (these may indicate sleep disordered breathing), assessment of the airway and appropriate investigations. Routine CXRs and ECGs are likely to be of poor quality and therefore of limited use.

Special equipment may be required for obese patients, including large gowns and stockings, blood pressure cuffs that are at least 20% greater than the diameter of the upper arm and operating tables that can accommodate the increased weight. Most operating theatre tables can take weights of approximately 130 kg, and the maximum weight should be labelled on each table, trolley and bed.[19]

Manual handling of the obese patient should be kept to a minimum and patients should be placed on the operating table prior to induction. The patient should be positioned with caution as areas may 'overhang' increasing the risk of contact with metal, slipping down the table in the head up position and pressure sores or nerve injuries. Extra gel pads, bean bags and supports should be available in theatre.

Venous thromboembolism (VTE) is a leading cause of death in obese patients and multi-modal VTE prophylaxis incorporating mechanical and pharmacological means is essential. Most hospitals will have evidence-based local protocols for VTE thromboprophylaxis.

DIABETES MELLITUS

Diabetes mellitus is the most common endocrine disease that surgeons will be faced with. Patients with Type 1 diabetes are treated with insulin, whereas those with Type 2 diabetes may start with diet and lifestyle modifications, but due to the progressive nature of the disease, are likely to eventually need oral hypoglycaemic agents and/or insulin.[20]

Patients with diabetes are at increased risk of complications such as hyperglycaemia, hypoglycaemia, diabetic ketoacidosis, postoperative surgical infections and perioperative mortality.[21] This risk can be minimised by good preoperative diabetic control as measured by glycated haemoglobin (upper limit 8–9%).

In general, the period of starvation for diabetic patients should be kept to a minimum, and this is best managed by placing them first on an operating list. All hospitals should have local protocols on how to manage diabetic medication, and clinicians should advise patients on individual adjustments whilst preparing for surgery.[22] Regular measurement of blood sugar is essential, aiming between 6 mmol/L and 10 mmol/L. In situations where the fasting period is prolonged, diabetic control is poor, or patients cannot resume their next meal, an insulin infusion may be required. This is now called 'variable rate intravenous insulin infusion', replacing the previously used term 'sliding scale' and uses 0.45% sodium chloride with 5% glucose and either 0.15% or 0.3% potassium chloride as the first choice for fluids.[22] Patients should resume their normal diabetic medication as soon as possible, usually when they have started to eat.

> **Key Point**
>
> Fasting times for patients with diabetes should be kept to a minimum and patients should be first on a list.

PERIOPERATIVE MANAGEMENT OF MEDICATION

In a study of 1,025 general surgical patients, Kennedy and colleagues reported that 49% of patients were taking medications unrelated to their surgical procedure and that these patients were at higher risk for a postoperative complication.[23] Whilst most chronic drugs are omitted on the day of surgery, there is a risk that 33% of them may not be restarted on the first postoperative day.[24] For many patients, this is because of ongoing fasting (40%), failure to represcribe (29%), drug withheld on doctor's orders (10%), drug unavailable in pharmacy or not as yet delivered to the ward (1%), or prolonged ileus (3%).[24] Of concern, 11.4% of elderly patients who had been taking warfarin continuously for at least 1 year did not resume their indicated warfarin therapy within 6 months after it was discontinued for elective in-patient surgery.[25]

In general, a thorough medication history is essential. Medications that have a withdrawal potential should be continued. Those medications that increase surgical risk should be stopped. Specific examples are listed in Table 1.5.

Key Point

Many medications can be continued perioperatively and can be taken with a sip of water upto 2 hours before surgery.

TABLE 1.5: Management of specific perioperative medication[26]

Medication	Comments
Diuretics, angiotensin-converting enzyme (ACE) inhibitors, angiotensin-receptor blockers	Omit on the morning of surgery because of risk of hypovolaemia/hypokalaemia
Beta-blockers, calcium-channel blockers	Continue at usual dose
Nonsteroidal anti-inflammatory drugs (NSAIDs)	May need to stop 1 week before depending on risk of bleeding during surgery
Digoxin	Should be continued and levels monitored if altered renal function
Central nervous system drugs—antiepileptics, antipsychotics, benzodiazepines, lithium, selective serotonin reuptake inhibitors, tricyclic antidepressants	These drugs have a significant potential for withdrawal and should be continued
Levodopa/carbidopa	Continue due to risk of deterioration of Parkinson's symptoms
Antithyroid drugs	Continue as there are no perioperative complications
Contraceptives	For major surgery with a prolonged period of immobilisation, stop 4 weeks before surgery due to increased risk of deep vein thrombosis (DVT). Alternatively, continue contraceptives and give higher intensity DVT prophylaxis
Methotrexate	Can increase the risk of wound infections and dehiscence. Many surgeons therefore withhold this drug for 1–2 weeks
Clopidogrel	Stop 7 days prior to surgery

ANTITHROMBOTIC THERAPY

The perioperative management of surgical patients taking warfarin is complicated and is based on an assessment of the risk of thromboembolism versus the risk of bleeding. Some procedures such as simple skin excisions and endoscopic procedures carry a low risk of bleeding, and it is therefore safe to continue anticoagulation. For procedures with a higher risk of bleeding such as neurosurgery, anticoagulation should be fully reversed aiming for an international normalised ratio (INR) of less than 1.3.[27]

Warfarin should be stopped 5 days before surgery, and the INR should be measured on the day of surgery. If the INR is greater than 1.5, then 1 mg of vitamin K can reduce the INR to a safe level, but may delay re-warfarinisation. If bridging therapy is required then either unfractionated heparin (UFH) or low molecular weight heparin (LMWH) should be started when the INR falls below the therapeutic range. Hospitals should have local guidelines on bridging regimes.

The last dose of LMWH should be administered 24 hours before surgery, whereas UFH has a short half-life and can be stopped 4 hours before surgery.[27] Instructions on when to resume bridging therapy must be communicated in the operation record and warfarin dosing guided using the Fennerty nomogram. In low-risk patients, warfarin can be restarted at the normal dose without the need for loading.

SAFE SURGERY

It is disappointing to learn that 45% of medical errors occur in the operating theatre and almost half of these are preventable.[28] The use of surgical safety checklists has been shown to decrease death rates from 1.5% to 0.8% and serious complications from 11% to 7%.[29]

The National Patient Safety Agency (NPSA) has launched an adaptation of the 2008 WHO surgical safety checklist, which is required for every patient undergoing surgery. Five steps to safer surgery involve the following:[30]
1. Briefing: Before the start of the list
2. Sign-in: Before the induction of anaesthesia and includes checking the patient's details and allergies
3. Timeout: Also known as the stop moment and takes place before the start of surgery
4. Sign-out: Before staff leave theatre, including steps such as the swab count
5. Debrief: At the end of the list to learn from incidents or address issues such as equipment failure.

Perceived benefits of the checklist are improved teamwork, improved safety, reduced near misses, smoother flow of procedures and better staff morale. However, the major obstacle to adoption of the checklist is a tendency to view the process as a tick box exercise with lack of clinical engagement.[30] Perhaps the greatest challenge to its adoption is a culture change amongst healthcare professionals.

> **Key Point**
>
> Implementation of the World Health Organization (WHO) surgical safety checklist reduces surgical complications and deaths.

PREOPERATIVE FASTING

This is defined as the period of time for which patients must refrain from any oral intake of liquids or solids before surgery to minimise the risk of pulmonary aspiration from gastric contents.

- Clear fluids such as water, fruit juices without pulp, carbonated beverages, clear tea and black coffee can be ingested upto 2 hours before surgery.
- A light meal and nonhuman milk (this behaves similar to solids in gastric emptying time) can be ingested 6 hours preoperatively.
- A fasting period of 8 hours is required for fried or fatty foods or meat.[31]

PERIOPERATIVE FLUID REPLACEMENT

All too often perioperative fluid replacement is left to the most junior member of the team who many not appreciate the subtleties of intravenous fluid therapy. Inadequate fluid replacement can lead to reduced oxygen delivery to tissues, including those that are injured, but too much fluid replacement can lead to acidosis, coagulation problems, and pulmonary and peripheral oedema. As with any other drug therapy, fluids have beneficial as well as side effects.

For most patients, fluids should be replaced orally with early resumption of food and drink. For patients who remain nil by mouth, fluids will need to be replaced intravenously, although studies have not confirmed whether crystalloids or colloids are superior (Table 1.6).[32]

TABLE 1.6: Commonly used crystalloids and colloids[32]

Crystalloids	Colloids
0.9% saline	Gelofusine
5% dextrose	Hetastarch
0.18% saline + 4% dextrose	Volulyte
Hartmann's solution	Human albumin 4.5%
Sodium bicarbonate 8.4%	

Another area that is often poorly considered is that of blood transfusion. There are many documented side effects associated with transfusion in surgical patients, such as increased risk of postoperative infection.[32] Hence, current guidelines recommend perioperative transfusion only when haemoglobin levels are below 70 g/L.

> **Key Point**
> Many patients do not need intravenous fluid therapy and should be encouraged to eat and drink as soon as possible after surgery.

PATIENT POSITIONING

Moving and positioning of the patient requires coordinated manual handling by the theatre team to avoid injury to staff and patients. There are many different surgical positions used to provide the best surgical access, whilst minimising risks to the patient (Table 1.7).

TABLE 1.7: Common surgical positions in theatre

Surgical position	Description
Supine	• Patients lie flat on their backs
	• Used for abdominal surgery
Lateral	• Patients lie on their side, often with a pillow between their knees
	• Used for hip/renal surgery
Prone	• Patients lie on their stomach with the chest supported to allow movement with respiration
	• Used for spinal/neurosurgery
Trendelenburg	• Patients lie flat on their backs with a head down position to allow the abdominal organs to move away from the pelvis
	• Used for lower abdominal or gynaecological surgery
Lithotomy	• Patients lie on their backs with their perineum at the edge of the operating table. Legs are often supported in stirrups.
	• Used for urological surgery
Lloyd-Davies	• Similar to lithotomy with legs apart and hips flexed
	• Used in colorectal and pelvic surgery

For any position, consideration should be given to avoid nerve/joint injuries, friction burns, damage to tissues, and prevention of patient slippage and pressure sores.

> **Key Point**
>
> Safe positioning of the patient requires good communication between the theatre team.

SUMMARY

Any patient's surgical journey is divided into three distinct phases, which are encompassed in the term perioperative care. The preoperative phase focuses on discussing the surgery, taking informed consent, and ensuring that resources are available for preassessment clinics. It is within the intraoperative phase that the patient is most vulnerable and totally reliant on the theatre team. It is therefore our priority that the patient comes to no harm with moving and surgical positioning, risk

> **Key Points**
>
> 1. Perioperative care incorporates the patient's entire surgical journey and includes pre-, peri- and postoperative care.
> 2. Preassessment clinics are essential to screen patients for fitness for an anaesthetic and surgery.
> 3. Laboratory tests should not be repeated for elective surgery if the results were normal within 4 months, providing there has been no change to the patient's condition.
> 4. Fasting times for patients with diabetes should be kept to a minimum and patients should be first on a list.
> 5. Many medications can be continued perioperatively and can be taken with a sip of water upto 2 hours before surgery.
> 6. Implementation of the World Health Organization (WHO) surgical safety checklist reduces surgical complications and deaths.

of infection, risk of DVT, and risk of hyper- or hypothermia. Postoperatively, our goals include managing the patient's pain, nausea and vomiting, and minimising surgical complications, whilst preparing

> 7. Many patients do not need intravenous fluid therapy and should be encouraged to eat and drink as soon as possible after surgery.
> 8. Safe positioning of the patient requires good communication between the theatre team.

the patient for prompt surgical discharge. Successful perioperative care, therefore, requires careful team work and communication at all times during this journey.

REFERENCES

1. http://www.dh.gov.uk/prod_consum_dh/groups/dh_digitalassets/@dh/@en/@ps/@sta/@perf/documents/digitalasset/dh_132599.xls
2. Niskanen MM, Takala JA. Use of resources and postoperative outcome. Eur J Surg. 2001;167(9):643-9.
3. Pearse RM, Harrison DA, James P, et al. Identification and characterisation of the high-risk surgical population in the United Kingdom. Crit Care. 2006;10(3):R81. Epub. 2006 Jun 2.
4. Pearse RM, Holt PJ, Grocott MP. Managing perioperative risk in patients undergoing elective noncardiac surgery. BMJ. 2011;343:d5759.
5. NHS Institute for Innovation and Improvement. Quality and Service Improvement Tools. [online] Available from http://www.institute.nhs.uk/option.com_quality_and_service_improvement_tools/Itemid,5015.html. [Accessed August 2012].
6. Findlay GP, et al. Knowing the risk. A review of perioperative care of surgical patients. NCEPOD 2011.
7. Bogod D. Consent. Ann R Coll Surg Engl. 2011;93(4):265-7.
8. Fitz-Henry J. The ASA classification and perioperative risk. Ann R Coll Surg Engl. 2011;93(3):185-7.
9. Kaplan EB, Sheiner LB, Boeckmann AJ, et al. The usefulness of preoperative laboratory screening. JAMA. 1985;253(24):3576-81.
10. Turnbull JM, Buck C. The value of preoperative screening investigations in otherwise healthy individuals. Arch Intern Med. 1987;147(6):1101-5.
11. Macpherson DS, Snow R, Lofgren RP. Preoperative screening: value of previous tests. Ann Intern Med. 1990;113(12):969-73.
12. Lopez-Argumedo M, Asua J. Preoperative evaluation in elective surgery. (INAHTA Synthesis Report). 1999. Osteba, Vitoria-Gasteiz. Dpt. of Health Basque Government. Basque Office for Health Technology Assessment.
13. National Institute for Clinical Excellence. Preoperative tests. The use of routine preoperative tests for elective surgery. London: NICE, 2003.
14. Velanovich V. The value of routine preoperative laboratory testing in predicting postoperative complications: a multivariate analysis. Surgery. 1991;109(3 Pt 1):236-43.
15. Noordzij PG, Boersma E, Bax JJ, et al. Prognostic value of routine preoperative electrocardiography on patients undergoing noncardiac surgery. Am J Cardiol. 2006;97(7):1103-6. Epub. 2006 Feb 28.

16. Archer C, Levy AR, McGregor M. Value of routine preoperative chest X-rays: a meta-analysis. Can J Anaesth. 1993;40(11):1022-7.
17. Sandler G. The importance of the history in the medical clinic and the cost of unnecessary tests. Am Heart J. 1980;106 (6 Pt 1):929-31.
18. Gohel MS, Bulbulia RA, Poskitt KR, et al. Avoiding blood transfusion in surgical patients (including Jehovah's Witnesses). Ann R Coll Surg Engl. 2011;93(6):429-31.
19. Reynolds N. Breathtaking obesity. Ann R Coll Surg Engl. 2011;93(5):339-42.
20. Game F. Update on drugs to treat diabetes. Ann R Coll Surg Engl. 2012;94:221-3.
21. Frisch A, Chandra P, Smiley D, et al. Prevalence and clinical outcome of hyperglycemia in the perioperative period in noncardiac surgery. Diabetes Care. 2010;33(8):1783-8.
22. Game F. Management of diabetes around emergency and elective procedures. Ann R Coll Surg Engl. 2012;94:293-6.
23. Kennedy JM, van Rij AM, Spears GF, et al. Polypharmacy in a general surgical unit and consequences of drug withdrawal. Br J Clin Pharmacol. 2000;49:353-62.
24. Kluger MT, Gale S, Plummer JL, et al. Perioperative drug prescribing pattern and manufacturers' guidelines. An audit. Anaesthesia. 1991;46(6):456-9.
25. Bell CM, Bajcar J, Bierman AS, et al. Potentially unintended discontinuation of long-term medication use after elective surgical procedures. Arch Intern Med. 2006;166:2525-31.
26. Whinney C. Perioperative medication management: general principles and practical applications. Cleve Clin J Med. 2009;76 (Suppl 4):S126-32.
27. Thapar A, Moore H, Golden D, et al. Perioperative antithrombotic therapy: bridging the gap. Ann R Coll Surg Engl. 2012;94:142-5.
28. Flin R, Yule S, McKenzie L, et al. Attitudes to teamwork and safety in the operating theatre. Surgeon. 2006;4:145-51.
29. Haynes AB, Weiser TG, Berry WR, et al. A surgical safety checklist to reduce morbidity and mortality in a global population. N Engl J Med. 2009;360:491-9.
30. Vickers R. Five steps to safer surgery. Ann R Coll Surg Engl. 2011;93(7):501-3.
31. Practice guidelines for preoperative fasting and the use of pharmacological agents for the prevention of pulmonary aspiration: application to healthy patients undergoing elective procedures. An updated Report to the American Society of Anaesthesiologists Committee on Standards and Practice Parameters. Anesthesiology. 2011;114:494-511.
32. Pearse RM, Ackland GL. Perioperative fluid therapy. BMJ. 2012;344:e2865.

2 | Biologic and Composite Mesh for Repair

Iain Anderson

Tissue repair is necessary to treat a range of conditions in general surgical practice, including groin hernias, incisional and parastomal hernias, hiatus hernia, recto-vaginal fistula and pelvic floor defects. It has long been recognised that suture repair alone is not always adequate and can lead to substantial recurrence rates,[1] and for over 150 years, surgeons have sought the ideal prosthetic implant. Advanced technologies have now provided biologic and composite meshes. Do these new categories of implant offer the ideal solution?

HISTORY

"If we could artificially produce tissues of the density and toughness of fascia and tendon, the secret of the radical cure of hernia would be discovered."

Billroth[1]

For years, surgeons have experimented with different prosthetic materials and these historic experiences remain pertinent. From the early 1800s, surgeons used gold wires followed by lead, aluminium, brass and silver coils on the floor of inguinal canal to buttress repair. This concept evolved into the use of hand-made filigrees but despite promising results with recurrence rates, their use faded due to lack of pliability resulting in patient discomfort, lack of inertness leading to fibrous reaction and the incidence of seromas, sinuses and infections.[2] Years later, stainless steel sutures were used in many anatomical locations and large series with long-term follow-up were published reporting excellent strength, durability, resistance to infection (0.1% infection rate) but difficulty of use limited the technique.[2] Tantalum (metallic) gauze became popular in the 1950s with little tissue reaction and few recurrences initially. However, with follow-up, later problems appeared with fatigue mesh fracture causing discomfort, recurrent herniation and difficulty in removing the prosthesis due to dense adhesions to underlying bowel.[2]

Synthetic polymers revolutionised suture and mesh materials. Nylon was used from the 1950s as a reliable suture material. Recurrence rates of 1.8-7.5% were reported with darn techniques but use of nylon net of any thickness was limited by infection.[2] Polyvinyl sponge (Ivalon®) faded out following reports of infection and disintegration with time.[2] These initial prosthetic meshes were followed by polyester and polypropylene and the latter inert monofilament mesh in particular, has been the mainstay of an era of tension-free repair and is still the most commonly used prosthesis. Modern meshes are tailored for shape, density and softness. These prosthetic materials have greatly reduced the incidence of recurrence rates following repair in a range of body sites and in some operations to less than 1%.[3]

This brief review of the history of prosthetics for repair has shown issues with infection, difficult handling, fatigue fracture, discomfort and difficulty with removal, and has emphasised the importance of adequate long-term follow-up of new techniques. Even successful modern monofilament meshes cause occasional complications with infection, adhesions, obstruction (5 to 11%) and bowel fistulas (3%).[4] Although uncommon in non-infected wounds, their occurrence can be disastrous and very difficult to treat. The predisposition to refractory infection stems from a nonbiological nature, and adhesions and fistulas from characteristics of the mesh which make it physically or biologically abrasive. These problems have led to the recent modification of synthetic mesh to yield composite implants which are less adherent. The search for an ideal implant especially in contaminated fields, where the risks of non-absorbable mesh become excessive, has led to the development of biologic implants.

> **Key Point**
>
> Conventional prosthetics are limited by chronic infection, adhesion to bowel causing obstruction and intestinal fistulation.

BIOLOGIC MESH

Biologic implants are derived from human (allograft) or animal (xenograft) sources and can be dermal or nondermal in origin (Table 2.1). Collagen-rich tissues such as skin, pericardium and intestinal submucosa are processed to remove all cellular components including DNA and major histocompatibility antigens. This reduces foreign body response. These tissues retain the natural 3D composition of the extracellular matrix (ECM), which acts as a tissue-remodelling scaffold into which the host cells can migrate and multiply.[5] The mesh components include growth factors which stimulate tissue regeneration and remodelling. The safety of some of the older bioscaffolds has been established from use in thousands of patients in many applications including tendon and ligament reconstruction, arterial grafts, stress urinary incontinence, augmentation cystoplasty, urethral and ureteral reconstruction, chronic ulcers, traumatic skin injury and nasal augmentation.

> **Key Point**
>
> Biologic meshes, derived from animal or human sources, act as scaffolds for native tissue and vascular in growth.

TABLE 2.1: Biologic mesh*

Source	Biologic mesh	Rehydration prior to use	Published human data (largest series)
Human dermis	Alloderm	20–30 min	n = 240[16]
Bovine pericardium	Periguard[X]	3 min	n = 7[51]
	Tutopatch	5–10 min	n = 29[29]
	Veritas	Not required	n = 30[31]
Foetal bovine dermis	SurgiMend	1 min	n = 0
Porcine small intestinal submucosa	Surgisis Gold	10 min	n = 133[21]
Porcine dermis	Collamend[X]	3 min	n = 25[9]
	Permacol[X]	Not required	n = 55[22]
	Strattice	2 min	n = 41[27]
	Xenmatrix	Not required	n = 57[52]

Keys: [X]: *Cross-linked; *: This is not an exhaustive list*

Structural Properties

Remodelling (native tissue and vascular in-growth into the implant and replacement of the implant with the host tissue) is a vital characteristic of these products, although the time points have not yet been accurately established in human studies and will likely differ between meshes. Some prostheses are subjected to collagen **cross-linking** by chemical treatment. This retards degradation by blocking collagenase-binding sites, and may enable the implant to maintain its structure for longer.

Animal studies have compared the host tissue in-growth and tensile strength between cross-linked and non cross-linked implants. One study compared four bioprostheses—Periguard, Permacol, Veritas and Alloderm. Permacol provided a strong and durable repair for upto 6 months. Periguard was equally strong but prone to infection and to skin ulceration. With time, Veritas and Alloderm had lost tensile strength associated with marked thinning; and with hernia-like bulging in the case of Alloderm.[6] Another study reported that non cross-linked porcine acellular dermal matrices were rapidly infiltrated with host cells[7] and vessels, whilst the cross-linked ones became encapsulated.[8] With encapsulation, cross-linked products may leave a bulkier scar; whether this is more resistant to recurrence (or alternatively a cause of later problems) is unknown. Fenestrations were shown to influence incorporation by allowing greater tissue incorporation without accelerating graft degradation.[9] The biologic meshes, certainly, differ in their thickness and handling characteristics. For example, cross-linked porcine dermal collagen (Permacol) is significantly thicker and tougher than the porcine submucosal collagen (Surgisis). Surgeons may have a preference for the handling characteristics of one type of product but as yet there are insufficient data to define the optimal usage profile of different biologics.

Human products need to be refrigerated whilst xenografts can be stored at room temperature. The shelf life of biologic meshes varies between 2–5 years and these implants require varied preparation before use such as rehydration ranging from 1–30 min (Table 2.1). Although this group of products is considered biocompatible, occasional severe foreign body reaction, and in one case mesh rejection has been reported. These products are harvested and processed carefully to ensure minimal risk of transmission of bacteria, viruses and prions, particular care being taken with products of bovine origin. Some manufacturers state that the transmission of infectious diseases may be ruled out at the level of the 'state of the art' only.

Importantly, biologic implants can be folded, cut or trimmed as required to fit the surgical site. They should be kept moist for which they should have tissue cover and maximum tissue contact is needed for integration. With drying or exposure of the implant, disintegration may occur but if rehydrated excessively, the product may soften too much and become unusable.

The cost of these biologics is very considerable and varies substantially from GBP 2 to 16 (USD 3.4 to 28) per cm^2. For comparison, the cost of commonly used polypropylene mesh is GBP 0.12 (USD 0.21) per cm^2. The porcine small intestine submucosa appears to be less expensive compared to the allografts, but given the relative paucity of evidence, the costs are very considerable. Biologic implants come in a range of sizes—a number of sheets sutured together can be required to repair large defects.

> **Key Point**
>
> Biologic meshes vary in structure and thickness with consequent differences in handling and immediate strength. However, the comparative clinical benefits remain unknown.

Clinical Use

The evidence for biologic meshes comes predominantly from retrospective case series. A potentially advantageous use for biologic meshes would be their use in contaminated and dirty wounds. However, the available literature shows that these products have been more commonly used in clean (Class I) and clean-contaminated (Class II) wounds. It is now promoted that for contaminated (Class III) and dirty (Class IV) wounds, biologic mesh offers a viable substitute to the patient's tissue, as they incorporate into native tissues and are considered resistant to infection. An animal study has illustrated the value of using biologics in Class III/IV wounds which demonstrated different rates of bacterial clearance (polyester synthetic 0%, Surgisis 58%, Permacol 67%, Xenmatrix 75%, and Strattice 92%) when these grafts were inoculated with *Staphylococcus aureus* in ventral hernia.[10]

Theoretically, if an implant was fully incorporated into native tissue, there should be no ongoing foreign body response and no scar formation. That could preclude the risk of chronic infection, erosion and fistulation. Adhesions to abdominal viscera have been claimed to be less with biologics, and some manufacturers have recommended direct placement over bowel. However, some authors have raised serious doubts over this based on observation from human series.[11] Manufacturers advise that if the patients require late re-operation, the site can be incised and closed using the same principles as for native tissue but experience is limited.

Remarkably, strong clinical evidence relating to the use of biologic implants is still in its early stages. Definitive studies have not yet appeared, and available evidence focuses mostly on abdominal wall reconstruction (AWR)—an area which we will use as an illustration. The term AWR in this literature refers to incisional and ventral hernia repair as well as much less common major complex reconstructions after fistulation and laparotomy. Obviously, the requirements of an implant under tension in an infected field are much greater than for one placed as an onlay in a non-infected field so extrapolating from one procedure to the next may not be adequate. Previously, some marketing strategies may not have made this clear.

Harth and Rosen reported major complications associated with xenografts in AWR from the Food and Drug Administration (FDA) database.[11] Although the total number of patients in which the xenografts were used has not been mentioned, 150 adverse events were identified of which 80% of implants were placed in an infected surgical field. These included acute mechanical failure, mesh disintegration, poor mesh integration, infection and fistulation. The majority of the adverse events occurred with cross-linked implants. Accurate delineation of the short- and long-term efficacy of biologics used in various clinical settings is still some way off and there is no conclusive evidence to differentiate between noncross-linked and cross-linked products in the human setting yet.

Allografts

Several human cadaveric grafts are available, of which Alloderm has been most used. AlloMax and FlexHD are other acellular human dermal implants but we are unaware of published human series.

Alloderm

This allogenic tissue graft, approved for use in 2002, has been used for burns, oral and abdominal wall defects, and to replace soft tissues in pelvic and plastic procedures. There is careful selection of donors to avoid disease transmission. It may be necessary to suture multiple sheets together to repair large defects. Post-operative diastasis can be a significant problem and may be secondary to inherent stretching of the mesh (upto 50%).[12] Table 2.2 gives a brief overview of evidence published for this product (all were open surgery). For comparison, repair with an open mesh technique with minimum follow-up of 12 months reported a 16.4% recurrence rate.[13]

A systematic review of 30 studies where acellular dermal matrix (Alloderm n = 26, Porcine n = 3, Bovine n = 1) was used in AWR showed an incidence of recurrent hernia ranging from 0 to 80%. Delayed wound healing occurred in upto 64% of patients. Infection-related complications including surgical site infections, cellulitis and deep/intra-abdominal abscesses were as high as 40%. Seroma was commonly reported and occurred in 27% of patients with human acellular dermal matrix.[14]

TABLE 2.2: Experience with Alloderm

Ist Author, Year	No. of patients	Class I+II/III+IV	Setting	Follow-up (months)	Complications
Patton, 2007[15]	67	0/67	AWR	10.6	Recurrence 18% SSC 24%
Diaz, 2009[16]	240	163/77	AWR	10.4	Recurrence 17%
					SSC 40%
					Fistula 12.6%
Lin, 2009[17]	144	123/21	Ventral hernia	5.8	Recurrence 27% SSC 37% Fistula 7.6% Mesh laxity 7.6%
Maurice and Skeete, 2009[18]	63	45/18	AWR	7.0	Recurrence 41% SSC 35%
Lee, 2009[19]	68	24/44	AWR	13.2+/-1.5	Recurrence 27% SSC 21% Dehiscence/ Evisceration 10% Fistula 10%

Abbreviations: *AWR: Abdominal wall reconstruction; SSC: Surgical site complications, i.e. infection, cellulitis, wound dehiscence, seroma, hematoma*

Porcine Xenografts

Among the xenografts, Surgisis and Permacol have the most studies published and probably the largest use to date in the UK. There is only one large series published for Xenmatrix. Periguard has one small human series and the FDA adverse events report published. SurgiMend has, as yet, no published human studies apart from the FDA adverse events report.

Surgisis

Surgisis is manufactured from small intestinal submucosa of pigs and was approved by the US FDA in 1999 for soft tissue repair. This product is available as four-layered (for para-oesophageal and groin hernia repair) and eight-layered products (for ventral hernia repair).

TABLE 2.3: Experience with Surgisis

Ist Author, Year	No. of patients	Class I+II/ III+IV	Setting	Open/ Lap	Follow-up (months)	Complications
Helton, 2005[20]	53	22/31	AWR	40/13	12–29	Recurrence 17% SSC 24%
Gupta, 2006[12]	41	38/3	Ventral hernia	41/0	29	SSC 41%
Franklin, 2008[21]	133	94/39	Mixed (inguinal, paraumbilical, incisional)	0/133	60	Recurrence 5% SSC 8% Pain 7%

Abbreviations: AWR: Abdominal wall reconstruction; Lap: Laparoscopic approach; SSC: Surgical site complications, i.e. infection, cellulitis, wound dehiscence, seroma, hematoma

Table 2.3 shows pooled published human data for Surgisis. Most were ventral hernia repairs and a few were inguinal hernia repairs. 40% were placed in a contaminated setting. The recurrence rates were between 5–30% (follow-up: 12–60 months). Surgisis has been placed at various tissue levels (onlay, sublay, inlay) and as interposition to bridge large defects. However, current recommendations do not advocate bridging: mesh incorporation is favoured by sublay or onlay. Presently, a double sandwich (sublay and onlay on either side of an abdominal wall closed by component separation) is recommended by the manufacturers.

Helton et al reported their experience of 53 abdominal wall reconstructions with Surgisis and found that use in dirty wounds in critically ill patients was associated with high complications, need for reoperation and recurrent hernia (39%) when compared with patients with clean and clean-contaminated wounds (9%).[20] The critically ill patients are the most challenging environment for any mesh but these findings suggest that biologic grafts do not necessarily provide a simple answer.

Permacol

Permacol is a decellularised, cross-linked, intact porcine dermal collagen. Table 2.4 summarises some published literature where Permacol has been used in AWR.

TABLE 2.4: Experience with Permacol

Ist Author, Year	No. of patients	Class I+II/ III+IV	Setting	Follow-up (months)	Complications
Cobb, 2005[22] (all laparoscopic)	55	51/4	Ventral hernia	14	Recurrence 7% SSC 4%
Shaikh, 2007[23] (all open)	20	15/5	AWR	18	Recurrence 15% SSC 35%
Hsu, 2008[24] (all open)	28	28/0	AWR	16	Recurrence 11% SSC 22%
Loganathan, 2010[25] (all open)	15	9/5	Incisional 10 Parastomal 4	12.6	Recurrence 13% Fistula 13%

Abbreviations: AWR: Abdominal wall reconstruction; SSC: Surgical site complications i.e. infection, cellulitis, wound dehiscence, seroma, hematoma

Permacol has also been used mostly in ventral hernias/complex AWR. This product has been used with open and laparoscopic repairs and is usually placed as an onlay or to bridge large defects. Although satisfactory short-term results have been reported, some authors highlight major concerns with cross-linked products including fistulation and dense adhesions.[11,25,26] Fistulation has been reported in 4 patients in the FDA report—with both cross-linked and non-cross-linked biologic meshes.[11] Recurrent fistulation occurred in 42% of patients who underwent reconstructive surgery for intestinal fistula in the open abdomen when Permacol was used.[26]

> **Key Point**
>
> Surgisis and Permacol, commonly used products in the UK, have shown reasonable short-term results in Class I/II cases; evidence in Class III/IV patients is as yet less convincing.

Strattice

This porcine dermal product was introduced relatively recently (2007). Acute mechanical failure was reported as one of the adverse events from the FDA database.[11] A retrospective review of 41 patients who underwent component separation with Strattice reinforcement for complex AWR has been reported with no hernia recurrence or symptomatic bulge after a mean follow-up period of 474 days. Strattice exposure occurred in 12.2% but there was no explantation.[27]

Collamend

This recent cross-linked porcine dermal product was used in 18 AWRs with reported recurrence of 44% and SSC of 39% at 7.3 months follow-up. Encapsulation was a major problem in cases with wound infection that required graft removal; hernia recurrence and dehiscence of the graft were problems even in non-compromised surgical fields.[28] The FDA database identified 25 adverse events associated with Collamend: acute mechanical failure/evisceration (n = 10), mesh disintegration (n = 2), poor mesh integration (n = 10), mesh infection (n = 2) and fistula (n = 1).[11]

Bovine Xenografts

Bovine pericardium meshes (Tutopatch, Veritas, Tutomesh) have a relative lack of elastin compared to dermal products (both allogenic and xenogenic). Some authors have suggested that this results in a higher ratio of mature collagen/elastin at the end of the remodelling, possibly minimising eventration and pseudo-recurrence. These products do not require refrigeration, have a long shelf life and can be used immediately after opening without long rehydration processes. They tend to be less expensive than allografts.

Tutopatch

Cattle are selected from 'closed herds' and deemed free of bovine spongiform encephalopathy. Tutopatch has been used in 29 neonates with gastroschisis and giant omphaloceles. These defects were repaired by primary closure (n = 5), onlay technique (n = 9) and bridged (n = 15). There were no recurrences reported at 2-year follow-up.[29]

Tutomesh

Two patients underwent complex AWR with Tutomesh placed in the retrorectus space and secured to the anterior abdominal wall using polypropylene sutures in a tension-free manner. There was no evidence of recurrence at 4- and 5-year follow-up.[30]

Veritas

The largest case series for this product was in 30 primary or recurrent ventral hernias treated in 26 patients with contaminated wounds or failure of a prosthetic mesh material. Veritas was placed as an inlay in 24 procedures: the recurrence rate was 19% with a mean follow-up of 22 months.[31] The FDA database reported 11 adverse events with this product in AWR—acute mechanical failure/evisceration (n = 7), mesh disintegration (n = 3) and other (n = 1).[11]

The data available for biologic implants are mostly retrospective case series or reports. There are no randomised clinical trials or even standardised prospective studies. Hence, it is difficult to draw conclusions especially regarding the choice and technique of the implant in what can be widely different settings. Although biologic implants were designed to be used in contaminated/dirty setting, most of the peer-reviewed publications have again been conducted in clean/clean-contaminated setting. Established biologic meshes appear safe, and although their effectiveness in challenging situations shows promise, this remains to be confirmed. The follow-up period of the above-mentioned studies have been short, and full evaluation of the longevity of these repairs is needed. Biologic meshes are expensive but some authors regard this as a logical and economical long-term solution which might reduce the need for two- or three-staged procedures. There is now a pressing need for comparative studies or at least data registries.

Parastomal Hernia Repair

Parastomal hernias can complicate upto 48% of stomas, and mesh repair has shown to achieve better results for this notoriously difficult abdominal wall hernia.[32] Even with prosthetic mesh repair, recurrence rates reach 33%.[33] One randomised controlled trial evaluated conventional stoma formation compared with the prophylactic use of a biologic mesh and reported significantly lower recurrence rates with the use of a mesh.[34] Other studies have reported comparable outcomes with biologic mesh repair (Table 2.5). On short-term follow-up, there have been no reports of mesh erosion or stenosis in these studies with biologic meshes.

TABLE 2.5: Studies using Biologic mesh for parastomal hernia repair

1st Author, Year	Mesh	No. of patients	Follow-up (months)	Complications
Hammond, 2008*[34]	Permacol (Sublay)	10	6.5	No recurrence/ complications (Recurrence 30% in controls)
Slater, 2011**[35]	Alloderm (Inlay, Onlay, under + Onlay sandwich) Periguard (Onlay) Surgisis (Sugarbaker)	57	8.1–50.2	Recurrence 15.7% Wound infection 5% Seroma 11%

Key: *: Randomised control trial; **: Systematic review of four studies*

One abdominal repair where randomised trial data support the use of biologic mesh relates to para-oesophageal hernia. A prospective randomised trial in 108 patients, reported significant improvement in recurrence rates at 6 months follow-up (Surgisis–9% vs Suture repair–24%). However, the second phase of this study at a median follow-up of 58 months demonstrated diminishing benefit in reducing hiatus hernia recurrence (Surgisis 54% vs Suture repair 59%).[36] Modest success with biologics has been reported in pelvic floor repair[37] and recto-vaginal fistula repair[38,39] where recurrence rates are high after surgical treatment, particularly in Crohn's disease, albeit on retrospective comparison.

COMPOSITE MESH

Composite meshes have been engineered to try and overcome the problems associated with non-absorbable synthetic meshes, especially adhesions and bowel erosion, whilst retaining the favourable properties of low recurrence rate, patient comfort and ease of handling.

Composite meshes are a combination of two different polymers, usually a non-absorbable mesh (typically polypropylene or polyester) with an anti-adhesive barrier, which is often absorbable. The absorbable barriers are designed to protect viscera from adhering to the permanent prosthetic long enough for the body to cover the mesh with a mesothelial layer. Most absorbable barriers degrade within 2 weeks, but the ideal duration of protection is unknown: neoperitonialisation may begin within 7 to 10 days according to some manufacturers. In a few, a non-adherent non-absorbable layer of ePTFE is used instead (Table 2.6).

Barriers can be on one or both sides. The former run the risk of exposing the bare prosthetic to the viscera along the edges. The latter have a theoretical risk of slowing abdominal wall tissue in-growth. Some authors report handling of some meshes to be easy laparoscopically attributing this to the softness of the absorbable barrier and the memory of the non-absorbable mesh.[40] Manufacturers advocate use of tacks ± non-absorbable sutures to margins of the mesh, but with some products this may expose the potentially adherent component.

TABLE 2.6: Commercially available** Composite mesh and their components

Composite mesh	Non-absorbable	Absorbable
C-Qur*	Polypropylene	Omega-3 fatty acid (both sides)
Composix Kugel	Polypropylene/ePTFE	None
Dulex	Polypropylene/ePTFE	None
Dynamesh*	Polypropylene	Polyvinylidene fluoride
Glucamesh*	Polypropylene	Beta-glucan
Intramesh T1	Polypropylene/ePTFE	None
Intramesh W3*	Polyester	Silicone
Parietene composite*	Polypropylene	Collagen
Parietex*	Polyester	Collagen
Proceed*	Polypropylene	Cellulose/polydioxanone
Sepramesh IR*	Polypropylene	Hydrogel

Keys: *: Coated mesh; **: Not an exhaustive list

Although composite meshes are still growing in popularity, there has been a reasonable number of case series published. Some 1092 open and 464 laparoscopic procedures have been reported (Table 2.7).

TABLE 2.7: Studies using composite mesh

Type	Author, Year	No. of patients	Setting	Follow-up (months)	Complications
Composix Kugel	Iannitti, 2008[41]	455 (open)	Ventral hernia (Recurrent 70%)	29.3	Recurrence 1.3% SSC 6.4%
	Cobb, 2009[42]	206 (open)	Ventral hernia		Infection 10.2%
Parietex	Balique, 2005[43]	80 (51–open; 29–lap)	Ventral hernia	48	Adhesions 14%
	Rosen, 2009[44]	79 (lap)	Ventral hernia	14	Infection 1% Bowel obstruction 1% (remote to mesh)
	Briennon, 2011[45]	280 (open)	Ventral hernia		Recurrence 3.2% Superficial infection 2% Deep infection 2% Seroma 5%
Proceed	Berrevoet, 2009[40]	114 (lap)	Ventral hernia	27	Chronic pain 1.8% Recurrence 3.5% Seroma 10.5%
	Moreno-Egea, 2009[46]	50 (20–open)	Incisional hernia	12	Nil

The cost of composite mesh varies depending on the dimensions and the anatomic repair it has been customised for. For example, Proceed mesh 15 × 15 cm costs GBP 300 (USD 480) and 20 × 30 cm costs GBP 700 (USD 1125), approximately. Unlike biologic meshes, pieces of composite meshes cannot usually be sutured together to cover large defects. Hence, the need arises to stock a costly range of varying sizes of mesh.

> **Key Point**
>
> Composite meshes are designed to be placed intraperitoneally and should be used in a Class I (clean) setting. Infection often requires removal.

Much of the composite mesh use has been driven by the desire to place a non-adherent mesh intraperitoneally by the laparoscope which is evident from the above studies. Clinical studies and preclinical animal models have attempted to determine the adhesion characteristics and effectiveness of barrier mesh prostheses.Studies have shown that composite mesh may have lower rate of adhesion formation: (18% versus 77%) when examined using ultrasound,[47] and 86% of patients were echographically free of adhesions 12 months after the intraperitoneal implantation of composite mesh.[43] Animal studies have shown that none of the coatings are completely able to prevent adhesions. A recent review has shown that Parietex and Dualmesh were cited most frequently for improvement of adhesion characteristics, followed closely by Sepramesh and C-QUR. Composix, Proceed and uncoated Polypropylene were cited most frequently as having the most tenacious and extensive adhesions.[47] It is unclear whether the source of adhesions is the mesh, the tacks or generalised scar response. Only one patient has reported to have developed small bowel fistula in relation to the mesh[49] but there have been case reports regarding mesh erosion/migration into bowel leading to enteric fistulation[50] and the authors are aware of others.

The consequences of mesh infection are very considerable due to the presence of non-absorbable component. Infection rates vary between 1–10%, and authors have raised concerns about MRSA infection—68% in one series.[49] In many cases, this will necessitate mesh removal: often a major undertaking. Chronic pain, which is a known complication of non-absorbable mesh, has been reported in a few studies ranging between 1.8% to as high as 30%.[40] Rates of late bowel obstruction are not available for these newer meshes to permit comparison with conventional ones (5 to 11%).[4]

Composite meshes possibly do offer advantage over non-absorbable meshes with respect to forming lesser adhesions but they have comparable recurrence rates and surgical site complications compared to conventional non-absorbable mesh. Their use is considered generally safe and effective in simple ventral hernias/AWR but they are expensive and complications such as bowel erosion and adhesions do occur. Long-term complication rates remain to be determined.

> **Key Point**
>
> Composite meshes have been reported to have comparable results with non-absorbable mesh with respect to recurrence and wound complication rates but fewer adhesions.

> **Key Points**
>
> 1. Conventional prosthetics are limited by chronic infection, adhesion to bowel causing obstruction and intestinal fistulation.
> 2. Biologic meshes, derived from animal or human sources, act as scaffolds for native tissue and vascular in-growth.
> 3. Biologic meshes vary in structure and thickness with consequent differences in handling and immediate strength. However, the comparative clinical benefits remain unknown.
> 4. Surgisis and Permacol, commonly used products in the UK, have shown reasonable short-term results in Class I/II cases; evidence in Class III/IV patients is as yet less convincing.
> 5. Composite meshes are designed to be placed intraperitoneally and should only be used in a Class I (clean) setting. Infection often requires removal.
> 6. Composite meshes have been reported to have comparable results with non-absorbable mesh with respect to recurrence and wound complication rates but fewer adhesions.

CONCLUSION

The development of Biologic and Composite meshes has brought exciting new prospects for tissue repair through attempting to overcome the risks and limitations of conventional polymer meshes. Each have their own advantages but all carry some disadvantages and most are very costly. As yet, most published data relate to case series rather than randomised controlled trials or prospective cohort studies. Most of the results have short- to medium-term follow-up. Hence until long-term studies and randomised controlled trials are available, these products should be used with consideration if not caution, and surgeons should audit their results openly. It may be that hybrid techniques such as modified component separation where a biologic/composite mesh is used to reinforce separated and spread host tissues will prove useful. Data are awaited.

REFERENCES

1. Read RC. Milestones in the history of hernia surgery: prosthetic repair. Hernia. 2004 Feb; 8(1):8-14.
2. DeBord JR. Protheses in hernia surgery: a century of evolution. In Bendavid R, Ed, Abdominal wall hernias: principles and management. 2001, Chapter 3, 16-32.
3. Lowham AS, Filipi CJ, Fitzgibbons RJ Jr, et al. Mechanisms of hernia recurrence after preperitoneal mesh repair. Traditional and laparoscopic. Ann Surg. 1997 Apr; 225(4):422-31. Review.
4. Leber GE, Garb JL, Alexander AI, et al. Long-term complications associated with prosthetic repair of incisional hernias. Arch Surg. 1998; 133:378–382.
5. Hodde J, Hiles M. Constructive soft tissue remodelling with a biologic extracellular matrix graft: overview and review of the clinical literature. Acta Chir Belg. 2007 Nov-Dec; 107(6):641-7.
6. Gaertner WB, Bonsack ME, Delaney JP. Experimental evaluation of four biologic prostheses for ventral hernia repair. J Gastrointest Surg. 2007 Oct; 11(10):1275-85.
7. de Castro Brás LE, Shurey S, Sibbons PD. Evaluation of crosslinked and non-crosslinked biologic prostheses for abdominal hernia repair. Hernia. 2012 Feb;16(1):77-89. Epub 2011 Jul 31.
8. Butler CE, Burns NK, Campbell KT, et al. Comparison of cross-linked and non-cross-linked porcine acellular dermal matrices for ventral hernia repair. J Am Coll Surg. 2010 Sep; 211(3):368-76.
9. Jenkins ED, Melman L, Deeken CR, et al. Evaluation of fenestrated and non-fenestrated biologic grafts in a porcine model of mature ventral incisional hernia repair. Hernia. 2010 Dec; 14(6):599-610.
10. Harth KC, Broome AM, Jacobs MR, et al. Bacterial clearance of biologic grafts used in hernia repair: an experimental study. Surg Endosc. 2011 Jul; 25(7):2224-9.
11. Harth KC, Rosen MJ. Major complications associated with xenograft biologic mesh implantation in abdominal wall reconstruction. Surg Innov. 2009 Dec; 16(4):324-9.
12. Gupta A, Zahriya K, Mullens PL, Salmassi S, Keshishian A. Ventral herniorrhaphy: experience with two different biosynthetic mesh materials, Surgisis and Alloderm. Hernia. 2006 Oct; 10(5):419-25.
13. den Hartog D, Dur AH, Tuinebreijer WE, Kreis RW. Open surgical procedures for incisional hernias. Cochrane Database Syst Rev. 2008 Jul; (3):CD006438.
14. Zhong T, Janis JE, Ahmad J, Hofer SO. Outcomes after abdominal wall reconstruction using acellular dermal matrix: a systematic review. Plast Reconstr Aesthet Surg. 2011 Dec; 64(12):1562-71.
15. Patton JH Jr, Berry S, Kralovich KA. Use of human acellular dermal matrix in complex and contaminated abdominal wall reconstructions. Am J Surg. 2007 Mar; 193(3):360-3.
16. Diaz JJ Jr, Conquest AM, Ferzoco SJ, et al. Multi-institutional experience using human acellular dermal matrix for ventral hernia repair in a compromised surgical field. Arch Surg, 144 (2009), pp. 209–215.

17. Lin HJ, Spoerke N, Deveney C, Martindale R. Reconstruction of complex abdominal wall hernias using acellular human dermal matrix: a single institution experience. Am J Surg. 2009 May; 197(5):599-603.

18. Maurice SM, Skeete DA. Use of human acellular dermal matrix for abdominal wall reconstructions. Am J Surg. 2009 Jan; 197(1):35-42.

19. Lee EI, Chike-Obi CJ, Gonzalez P, et al. Abdominal wall repair using human acellular dermal matrix: a follow-up study. Am J Surg. 2009 Nov; 198(5):650-7.

20. Helton WS, Fisichella PM, Berger R, et al. Short-term outcomes with small intestinal submucosa for ventral abdominal hernia. Arch Surg. 2005 Jun; 140(6):549-62.

21. Franklin ME Jr, Treviño JM, Portillo G, et al. The use of porcine small intestinal submucosa as a prosthetic material for laparoscopic hernia repair in infected and potentially contaminated fields: long-term follow-up. Surg Endosc. 2008 Sep; 22(9):1941-6.

22. Cobb GA, Shaffer J. Cross-linked acellular porcine dermal collagen implant in laparoscopic ventral hernia repair: case-controlled study of operative variables and early complications. Int Surg. 2005 Jul-Aug; 90(3 Suppl):S24-9.

23. Shaikh FM, Giri SK, Durrani S, Waldron D, Grace PA. Experience with porcine acellular dermal collagen implant in one-stage tension-free reconstruction of acute and chronic abdominal wall defects. World J Surg. 2007 Oct; 31(10):1966-75.

24. Hsu PW, Salgado CJ, Kent K, et al. Evaluation of porcine dermal collagen (Permacol) used in abdominal wall reconstruction. J Plast Reconstr Aesthet Surg. 2009 Nov; 62(11):1484-9.

25. Loganathan A, Ainslie WG, Wedgwood KR. Initial evaluation of Permacol bioprosthesis for the repair of complex incisional and parastomal hernias. Surgeon. 2010 Aug; 8(4):202-5.

26. Connolly PT, Teubner A, Lees NP, et al. Outcome of reconstructive surgery for intestinal fistula in the open abdomen. Ann Surg. 2008 Mar; 247(3):440-4.

27. Patel KM, Nahabedian MY, Gatti M, Bhanot P. Indications and Outcomes following complex abdominal reconstruction with component separation combined with porcine acellular dermal matrix reinforcement. Ann Plast Surg. 2011 Dec 9. [Epub ahead of print]

28. Chavarriaga LF, Lin E, Losken A, et al. Management of complex abdominal wall defects using acellular porcine dermal collagen. Am Surg. 2010 Jan; 76(1):96-100.

29. van Tuil C, Saxena AK, Willital GH. Experience with management of anterior abdominal wall defects using bovine pericard. Hernia. 2006 Mar; 10(1):41-7.

30. Cavallaro A, Lo Menzo E, Di Vita M, et al. Use of biological meshes for abdominal wall reconstruction in highly contaminated fields. World J Gastroenterol. 2010 Apr 21; 16(15):1928-33.

31. Limpert JN, Desai AR, Kumpf AL, Fallucco MA, Aridge DL. Repair of abdominal wall defects with bovine pericardium. Am J Surg. 2009 Nov; 198(5):e60-5.

32. Carne PW, Frye JN, Robertson GM, Frizelle FA. Parastomal hernia following minimally invasive stoma formation. ANZ J Surg. 2003 Oct; 73(10):843-5. Review.

33. Tam KW, Wei PL, Kuo LJ, Wu CH. Systematic review of the use of a mesh to prevent parastomal hernia. World J Surg. 2010 Nov; 34(11):2723-9.

34. Hammond TM, Huang A, Prosser K, Frye JN, Williams NS. Parastomal hernia prevention using a novel collagen implant: a randomised controlled phase 1 study. Hernia. 2008 Oct; 12(5):475-81.

35. Slater NJ, Hansson BM, Buyne OR, Hendriks T, Bleichrodt RP. Repair of parastomal hernias with biologic grafts: a systematic review. J Gastrointest Surg. 2011 Jul; 15(7):1252-8.

36. Oelschlager BK, Pellegrini CA, Hunter JG, et al. Biologic prosthesis to prevent recurrence after laparoscopic paraesophageal hernia repair: long-term follow-up from a multicenter, prospective, randomized trial. J Am Coll Surg. 2011 Oct; 213(4):461-8

37. Wahed S, Ahmad M, Mohiuddin K, Katory M, Mercer-Jones M. Short-term results for laparoscopic ventral rectopexy using Biologic mesh for pelvic organ prolapse. Colorectal Dis. 2011 Dec 18. doi: 10.1111/j.1463-1318.2011.02921.x. [Epub ahead of print]

38. Ellis CN. Outcomes after repair of rectovaginal fistulas using bioprosthetics. Dis Colon Rectum. 2008 Jul; 51(7):1084-8.

39. Schwandner O, Fuerst A, Kunstreich K, Scherer R. Innovative technique for the closure of rectovaginal fistula using Surgisis mesh. Tech Coloproctol. 2009 Jun; 13(2):135-40.

40. Berrevoet F, Fierens K, De Gols J, et al. Multicentric observational cohort study evaluating a composite mesh with incorporated oxidized regenerated cellulose in laparoscopic ventral hernia repair. Hernia. 2009 Feb; 13(1):23-7.

41. Iannitti DA, Hope WW, Norton HJ, et al. Technique and outcomes of abdominal incisional hernia repair using a synthetic composite mesh: a report of 455 cases. J Am Coll Surg. 2008 Jan; 206(1):83-8.

42. Cobb WS, Carbonell AM, Kalbaugh CL, Jones Y, Lokey JS. Infection risk of open placement of intraperitoneal composite mesh. Am Surg. 2009 Sep; 75(9):762-8.

43. Balique JG, Benchetrit S, Bouillot JL, et al. Intraperitoneal treatment of incisional and umbilical hernias using an innovative composite mesh: four-year results of a prospective multicenter clinical trial. Hernia. 2005 Mar; 9(1):68-74.

44. Rosen MJ. Polyester-based mesh for ventral hernia repair: is it safe? Am J Surg. 2009 Mar; 197(3):353-9.

45. Briennon X, Lermite E, Meunier K, Desbois E, Hamy A, Arnaud JP. Surgical treatment of large incisional hernias by intraperitoneal insertion of Parietex® composite mesh with an associated aponeurotic graft (280 cases). J Visc Surg. 2011 Feb; 148(1):54-8.

46. Moreno-Egea A, Aguayo-Albasini JL, Ballester MM, Cases Baldó MJ. Treatment of incisional hernias adopting an intra-abdominal approach with a new low-density composite prosthetic material: proceed: our preliminary experience on 50 cases. Surg Laparosc Endosc Percutan Tech. 2009 Dec; 19(6):497-500.

47. Arnaud JP, Hennekinne-Mucci S, Pessaux P, Tuech JJ, Aube C. Ultrasound detection of visceral adhesion after intraperitoneal ventral hernia treatment: a comparative study of protected versus unprotected meshes. Hernia. 2003 Jun; 7(2):85-8.

48. Deeken CR, Faucher KM, Matthews BD. A review of the composition, characteristics, and effectiveness of barrier mesh prostheses utilized for laparoscopic ventral hernia repair. Surg Endosc. 2012 Feb; 26(2):566-75.

49. Cobb WS, Harris JB, Lokey JS, McGill ES, Klove KL. Incisional herniorrhaphy with intraperitoneal composite mesh: a report of 95 cases. Am Surg. 2003 Sep; 69(9):784-7.

50. Nelson EC, Vidovszky TJ. Composite mesh migration into the sigmoid colon following ventral hernia repair. Hernia. 2011 Feb; 15(1):101-3.

51. Zardo P, Zhang R, Wiegmann B, Haverich A, Fischer S. Biological materials for diaphragmatic repair: initial experiences with the PeriGuard Repair Patch®. Thorac Cardiovasc Surg. 2011 Feb; 59(1):40-4.

52. Byrnes MC, Irwin E, Carlson D, et al. Repair of high-risk incisional hernias and traumatic abdominal wall defects with porcine mesh. Am Surg. 2011 Feb; 77(2):144-50.

3 Perioperative Cardiopulmonary Exercise Testing for Major Abdominal Surgery

Malcolm West, Sandy Jack, Michael PW Grocott

INTRODUCTION

Major abdominal surgery is associated with a substantial burden of postoperative morbidity and mortality particularly in elderly patients and those with co-morbidities. Recent national audits in the UK have documented 30-day mortality rates of 2.3% for elective colon cancer surgery,[1] 2.6% for elective rectal cancer surgery, 7.3% for elective aortic surgery,[2] 4.0% for elective oesophageal and gastric surgery (78% 1-year survival)[3] and 11.4% for emergency colonic surgery.[1] It has been estimated that more than 4 million surgical procedures are performed annually in the UK, 12.3% of which are performed on patients classified as "high-risk" (expected mortality > 5%). In this analysis, the "high-risk" group accounted for the majority of postoperative mortality (83.4%), and had a significantly longer hospital stay and therefore increased resource usage.[4] Outcome after major surgery is dependent on modifiable factors, such as the medical care received before, during and after surgery, as well as more fixed factors, such as the patient's physiological tolerance of surgical trauma. Accurate risk prediction allows the multidisciplinary team to ensure appropriate modification of patients' preoperative status as well as optimising intra- and postoperative management for high-risk surgical patients. Such risk prediction also facilitates the most efficient use of scarce resources (e.g. intensive care beds). Importantly, better risk prediction also provides a higher quality of data to physicians and patients to enhance the process of shared decision making before surgery.[5] The preoperative identification of patients at high risk of adverse outcome following the trauma of major surgery should be a priority. A variety of approaches to risk evaluation has been proposed including clinical acumen, clinical prediction scores [American Society of Anesthesiologists (ASA), Duke's Activity Scores, Physiological and Operative Severity Score for the enUmeration of Mortality and Morbidity (POSSUM), colorectal specific POSSUM (CR-POSSUM), etc.],[6-8] plasma biomarkers[9] and various measures of cardiac function.[10-12] Evaluating exercise tolerance using shuttle walk tests[13-15] or cardiopulmonary exercise testing (CPET) has been used extensively for risk prediction before thoracic or abdominal surgery. Whilst the relationship between the simpler measures of exercise tolerance (e.g. stair climbing, shuttle walk tests) and CPET is known to be relatively weak,[16,17] the comparative performance of these different approaches in predicting perioperative risk is currently uncertain due to the paucity of available data. Cardiopulmonary exercise testing utilising breath-by-breath expired gas analysis is currently the most objective and precise means of evaluating physical fitness prior to surgery. This review will focus on the application of CPET to preoperative risk prediction for major abdominal surgery.

CARDIOPULMONARY EXERCISE TESTING

Almost two decades ago, Older and colleagues identified an association between low functional capacity (low fitness levels) as determined by CPET, and poor patient outcome following non-cardiopulmonary surgery.[18] Based on this and subsequent published literature, CPET-derived variables have been increasingly adopted as the objective measures of fitness prior to surgery, particularly within the National Health Service (NHS) in the UK.[19] Information derived from CPET is now used to inform operative decisions, choice of peri- and intraoperative management as well as to inform discussion of operative risk with patients.[7] This chapter aims to provide a basic understanding of the physiological assessments carried out when performing a CPET and to review the current literature pertaining to the value of CPET as a tool to evaluate perioperative risk and thereby improve the management of patients undergoing major abdominal surgery.

> **Key Point**
>
> Risk prediction from CPET should always be evaluated in the context of the overall clinical picture.

Cardiopulmonary exercise testing is a well tolerated, noninvasive, cost-effective way to perform perioperative risk assessment in patients who are scheduled to undergo high-risk procedures. It is also useful for those who are at high risk of postoperative complications due to advanced age or poor nutritional status, and for those with a history of cardiopulmonary morbidity. It provides a global assessment of the integrated response to increasing aerobic work involving the cardiovascular, respiratory, neuropsychological and skeletal muscle systems, all of which are activated during the metabolic stress response to surgery.[20] It allows evaluation of the integrated oxygen delivery system when the demand for oxygen is high and the system is required to function near to its maximum capacity. Despite requiring a moderate to high level of exertion, CPET is well tolerated by patients[21,22] and is safe to conduct on most patient cohorts.[23] The data from CPET, including oxygen uptake at peak exercise (peak VO_2), the anaerobic threshold or lactate threshold (AT/LT), oxygen pulse (O_2 pulse at LT) and ventilatory equivalent (V_E/VCO_2 at LT) predict morbidity and mortality in the perioperative

> **Key Point**
>
> Cardiopulmonary exercise testing can be used for risk stratification and perioperative patient management.

period,[24] as well as being independent predictors of occult heart and lung disease.

Conduct of a Cardiopulmonary Exercise Testing

In the assessment of preoperative risk, CPET is usually conducted on an electromagnetically-braked cycle ergometer with the patient breathing through a mouthpiece or facemask through which gas exchange is measured. The patient is also monitored using a continuous 12-lead ECG and oxygen saturation, and periodic measurement of blood pressure. A typical CPET set-up is shown in Figure 3.1. Common CPET variables and their definitions are detailed in Table 3.1. The test protocol normally includes four phases: an initial rest phase (approximately 3 minutes) is employed to establish baseline values, followed by an unloaded cycling (zero watts) phase to allow the patient to become familiar with the cycling motion and to reduce the influence of the lag present between increased work rate (WR) and the

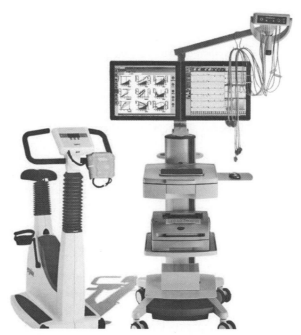

Figure 3.1: CPET set-up including metabolic cart, bike, ECG, etc

oxygen uptake (VO_2) response.[25] Following this, the incremental exercise phase begins. A ramp protocol is commonly used, during which the set WR is increased linearly with time, with a corresponding increase in the intensity of the exercise. The ramp incremental protocol can be determined by using a formula by Wasserman and colleagues:[25]

$$VO_2 \text{ unloaded pedalling (mL/min)} = 150 + (6 \times \text{weight in kg})$$
$$\text{Peak } VO_2 \text{ (mL/min)} = \text{Height (cms)} - \text{Age (years)} \times 20 \text{ (sedentary males)}$$
$$\text{Peak } VO_2 \text{ (mL/min)} = \text{Height (cms)} - \text{Age (years)} \times 14 \text{ (sedentary females)}$$
$$\text{Work rate increment/min} = \text{Peak } VO_2 - VO_2 \text{ unloaded pedalling/100}$$

TABLE 3.1: Cardiopulmonary exercise testing (CPET) variable definitions

CPET variables	Definitions
Lactate or anaerobic threshold (LT or AT)	The exercise VO_2 above which anaerobic high-energy phosphate production supplements aerobic high-energy phosphate production, with consequential lowering of the cellular redox state, increase in lactate/pyruvate (L/P) ratio, and net increase in lactate production at the site of anaerobiosis. Exercise above the AT is reflected in the muscle effluent and central blood by an increase in lactate concentration, L/P ratio and metabolic acidosis.
Heart rate reserve (HRR)	The difference between the predicted highest heart rate attainable during maximum exercise and the actual highest heart rate.
Maximal oxygen uptake ($VO_{2\,max}$)	Describes the VO_2 when it reaches a plateau value during a single maximum work rate (WR) test. Repeated measurements necessary to obtain the VO_2 that cannot be exceeded by the subject.
Oxygen pulse (O_2 pulse)	The oxygen uptake (VO_2) divided by the heart rate. Hence, this represents the amount of oxygen extracted by the tissue of the body from the O_2 carried in each stroke volume.
Oxygen uptake (VO_2)	The amount of oxygen extracted from the inspired gas in a given period of time, expressed in mL or L per minute.
Peak oxygen uptake (VO_2 peak)	The highest VO_2 achieved during a maximum work rate test.
Work rate (WR)	The rate at which work is preformed in watts.
Ventilatory equivalents for CO_2 and O_2 (VE/VCO_2 and VE/VO_2)	The ventilatory equivalents for CO_2 and O_2 are measurements of the ventilatory requirement for a given metabolic rate.
Minute ventilation (VE)	The volume of gas exhaled divided by the time of collection in minutes.

The criteria for test termination differ between laboratories; in some, the test is terminated by the patient at volitional exhaustion or symptoms (e.g. shortness of breath, chest pain, etc.), whilst others perform a submaximal test and stop exercise when a particular criterion is met, such as a respiratory exchange ratio (RER) above 1.[22] However, this is not felt to be a reliable indication of LT due to the interaction of hyperventilation. One should aim for an exercise period between 8 minutes and 12 minutes. Following test completion, a recovery period of low intensity exercise should be performed to maintain venous return, thereby reducing the risk of pooling of blood in the leg veins, which can be associated with symptomatic hypotension (e.g. light-headedness, faint). The patient should be observed throughout recovery until physiological variables, including heart rate, blood pressure, ventilation and oxygen saturation, have returned close to baseline levels and any exercise induced ECG changes have resolved. The test should be stopped if the patient experiences any adverse symptoms (Table 3.2).[23,26,27]

TABLE 3.2: Adverse indications for stopping cardiopulmonary exercise testing (CPET)

• Angina
• > 2 mm ST depression if symptomatic or 4 mm if asymptomatic or > 1 mm ST elevation
• Significant arrhythmias
• Fall in systolic pressure > 20 mmHg from the highest value during the test
• Hypertension > 250 mmHg systolic; > 120 mmHg diastolic
• Severe desaturation: SpO_2 < 80% accompanied by limiting hypoxaemia
• Sudden pallor
• Loss of coordination
• Mental confusion
• Signs of respiratory failure

Cardiopulmonary Exercise Testing-Derived Variables

A number of different physiological variables are measured or derived (Table 3.2) when performing a CPET. Some of these variables have been used to identify patients at high risk of perioperative morbidity and mortality: estimated LT,[18,21,22,28] peak VO_2[29] and V_E/VCO_2.[22,30] Consequently, these three variables are most commonly used to stratify risk for non-cardiopulmonary surgery.[19,24,31-33]

As WR increases, VO_2 and VCO_2 increase linearly until the point at which lactic acidosis develops. This changing relationship can be used to identify the LT using a technique known as the "V-slope" method.[25,34] VCO_2 is plotted against VO_2 with the former on the y-axis and the latter on the x-axis. The two variables will rise at the same rate before the ventilatory threshold and a best-fit line through these points will have a slope close to 1. At WR above the LT, CO_2 output increases more rapidly than O_2 uptake (slope is greater than 1) because CO_2 generated by the bicarbonate buffering of lactic acid is added to the metabolic CO_2 production. The intercept of these two slopes is the estimated LT as measured by gas exchange (Fig. 3.2).

The modified V-slope method identifies the LT as the tangential breakpoint in the VCO_2-VO_2 relationship from the line of unity ("line of one") during the incremental stage of the exercise test (Fig. 3.3). The V-slope methods depend solely on the physicochemical reaction of lactate with bicarbonate and

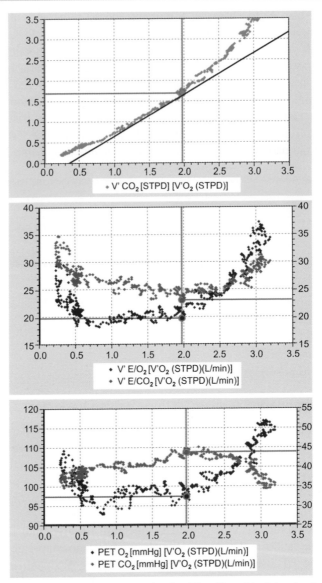

Figure 3.2: An example trace showing LT and how it is determined

as such the occurrence of the breakpoint is independent of chemoreceptor sensitivity and the ventilatory response to exercise, although the magnitude of the response is dependent on these factors.[34,35] Whilst the physiological basis for this variable remains controversial,[36] the interobserver variability for experienced clinicians is very acceptable.[37] The LT is therefore regarded as an effort independent, submaximal exercise marker of the adequacy of oxygen delivery to the metabolising muscle and is usually more than 40% of the predicted peak VO_2, making it an important marker of cardiopulmonary

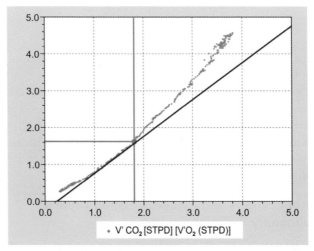

Figure 3.3: The modified V-slope method of AT determination. At the anaerobic threshold the gradient of the VO_2-VCO_2 relationship will increase above 1. The breakpoint—marked by the green vertical line is the AT

fitness.[24,25] The LT compliments other very important information derived from the whole exercise test and should not be taken as a single variable in isolation.

Other important variables derived from CPET are peak VO_2, V_E/VCO_2 and V_E/VO_2. Peak VO_2 is the highest VO_2 achieved during CPET and generally occurs at or near peak exercise, which is calculated from the averaged last 30 seconds of data. Peak VO_2 is another useful measure of aerobic capacity and is related to age, sex, weight and type of work performed. A formula for estimating peak VO_2 reported by Wasserman and Whipp[25] is as follows:

Predicted VO_2 during unloaded pedalling (mL/min) = $(5.8 \times$ weight in kg$) + 151$

Peak VO_2 (mL/min) = Height (cm) – age (years) $\times$ 20 (sedentary males) or $\times$ 14 (sedentary females)

Moreover, if the VO_2 curve demonstrates a plateau, such that the VO_2 no longer increases despite progressive increments in workload, then the peak VO_2 can also be labelled as the VO_{2max}. VO_{2max} is the best and most reproducible index of cardiopulmonary fitness or disability, but is very difficult to achieve in the preoperative setting.[25]

The major link between the circulation and ventilatory responses to exercise is CO_2 production. The breathing requirements of exercise can be described from the following equation:

$$V_E = \frac{863 \cdot VCO_2}{PaCO_2 \cdot (1 - V_D/V_T)}$$

or

$$V_E = \frac{863 \cdot VO_2 \cdot R}{PaCO_2 \cdot (1 - V_D/V_T)}$$

in which $PaCO_2$ is the set point and controller and ventilation increases with VCO_2 as a frame of reference. V_E/VCO_2 is the respiratory control function that reflects chemoreceptor sensitivity, acid-base balance and ventilator efficiency at the alveolar-capillary interface.

For more detailed descriptions of CPET protocols and physiology, the reader is directed to the American Thoracic Society/American College of Chest Physicians statement on CPET[23] and Principles of Exercise Testing by Wasserman and colleagues.[25]

Current Applications and Evidence-Based Value of Cardiopulmonary Exercise Testing

In his seminal early study, Older and colleagues showed that cardiovascular mortality was virtually restricted to patients with an LT of less than 11 mL/kg/min.[18] Since this publication in the early 1990s, a large number of studies have addressed the association between CPET-derived variables and perioperative outcome in a variety of clinical contexts. Several of these have also evaluated the predictive utility of CPET-derived variables as a means of describing perioperative risk in clinical practice. The next section reviews this literature to evaluate the utility of CPET as a risk stratification tool prior to major (mainly abdominal) surgery.

> **Key Points**
>
> - Specific CPET-derived variables seem to have particular predictive value for specific surgical types.
> - In general, a prudent approach, characterised by conservative estimation of perioperative risk, is likely to result in optimal patient outcomes, but this needs to be balanced against the increased resource usage (e.g. ICU bed days).

Major Intra-Abdominal Surgery

Older and colleagues[18] recorded the presurgical LT of 187 elderly patients undergoing major intra-abdominal surgery. They found that an LT less than 11mL/kg/min was associated with increased cardiovascular mortality. In patients with a low LT and preoperative ischaemia, the mortality rate was 42%, in comparison with 4% in patients not meeting these criteria. This established the idea of preoperative risk stratification and provision of increased postoperative care for high-risk patients. In a latter study and clinical review,[28,38] Older investigated the impact of triaging patients on the basis of such data. If a patient had an LT of less than 11mL/min/kg, they were assigned to ICU preoperatively. This accounted for 28% of the patients. Of the 9 patients who died postoperatively from cardiopulmonary complications, 7 had an LT less than 11 mL/min/kg, and the other two were in the high dependency units (HDU) category. No deaths were recorded in the ward admissions.

Assessing 843 patients undergoing major colorectal surgery, radical nephrectomy and cystectomy, Wilson and colleagues[22] concluded that in this patient cohort (aged > 55 years), an LT of 10.9 mL/kg/min or less and a V_E/VCO_2 of 34 or more had a sensitivity of 88% and a specificity of 47% for hospital mortality. Survival at 90 days was significantly greater in patients with an AT of greater than 11 (p = 0.034), V_E/VCO_2 less than 34 (p = 0.021) and in patients without ischaemic heart disease (p = 0.02). Snowden and colleagues[21] also evaluated the use of CPET in preoperative risk assessment in a surgical population (age mean 70 years). They reported the relationship between CPET-derived variables and morbidity after major intra-abdominal surgery and showed that an LT of 10.1 mL/kg/min had the optimal values of sensitivity (88%) and specificity (79%) for the prediction of postoperative complications, determined by receiver operating characteristic (ROC) curve analysis. In a smaller study in 32 patients undergoing major intra-abdominal surgery, Hightower and colleagues[6] reported that an LT less than 75% of the predicted value identified those at increased risk of complications [area under curve (AUC) 0.72; sensitivity 88%; specificity 79%; p = 0.016].

A particular strength of the studies by Snowden and Hightower is that clinicians were blinded to the CPET results, ensuring that these did not influence patient care or data collection. This should give a more accurate reflection of the true magnitude of association between CPET variables and outcome by removing the effect of confounding due to clinicians acting on CPET variables, which could and influence outcome (e.g. choice of level of postoperative care received by the patient).[39]

In a recent publication, Junejo and colleagues[40] evaluated the use of preoperative CPET in predicting outcome following major hepatic resection. Two hundred and four patients were assessed for hepatic resection, of whom 108 had preoperative CPET. An LT of 9·9 mL/kg/min predicted in-hospital death and subsequent survival. Below this value, LT was 100% sensitive and 76% specific for in-hospital mortality. Age and V_E/VCO_2 at LT (34.6 = 84% specificity and 47% sensitivity) were also significantly related to postoperative complications. Long-term survival of those with a LT of less than 9·9 mL/kg/min was significantly worse [Hazard ratio for mortality 1·81, 95% confidence interval (CI), 1·04–3·17; p = 0·036].

In summary, all the above studies agree that LT and V_E/VCO_2 at LT have a predicative value in determining postoperative complications across a range of surgical procedures.

> **Key Point**
>
> An LT of 11 mL/kg/min appears to be an acceptable threshold to use in a clinical setting to indicate increased perioperative risk following major intra-abdominal surgery, despite some indication that this value may lower in some centres.

Vascular Surgery

Nugent et al[41] highlighted the potential use of CPET for identifying high-risk individuals prior to undergoing an abdominal aortic aneurysm (AAA) repair in an elderly population (mean age 72 years). Based on this small study (30 patients), the authors advocate that a peak VO_2 of less than 20 mL/kg/min as a marker of patients at increased perioperative risk, despite no differences in peak VO_2 being present between patients with or without postoperative complications. Following this, Carlisle and Swart[30] retrospectively studied the association between four CPET markers (peak VO_2, LT, V_E/VCO_2 and V_E/VO_2), four other risk stratification methods [revised cardiac risk index (RCRI), POSSUM, simplified acute physiology score (SAPS) II and the acute physiology and chronic health evaluation (APACHE) II] and all-cause mortality following abdominal aortic aneurysm (AAA) repair. The study differs from other CPET articles in non-cardiopulmonary surgery, in that the mortality was not only measured in the initial postoperative period, but also up to a median of 35 months, termed mid-term. Of the 130 patients studied, a total of 29 (22.3%) had died by the time of the last follow-up, 14 (10.8%) doing so in hospital within 30 days of surgery. All CPET variables correlated with mid-term survival, as did the other four risk stratification methods, although to a lesser degree. The V_E/VCO_2 had the strongest association with mortality rate at 30 days and at mid-term, when the hazard ratio for mortality was 1.14 (95% CI, 1.08–1.20; p < 0.001). Of the perioperative risk scores, the RCRI had the strongest association with survival with a hazard ratio of 1.86 (95% CI, 1.25–2.78; p = 0.002). A V_E/VCO_2 value of greater than or equal to 42 and RCRI greater than 1 were found to be the optimal thresholds to distinguish patients at increased risk of death. In summary, both studies suggest that there is a weak relationship between peak VO_2 and postoperative morbidity and mortality in patients undergoing elective AAA repair. Only Carlisle and colleagues found the role of LT to be a strong predictor.

> **Key Point**
>
> A V_E/VCO_2 greater than or equal to 42 should be used to help identify high-risk patients undergoing AAA repair surgery; however, hyperventilation should always be considered as this can artificially inflate this variable.

Upper Gastrointestinal and Bariatric Surgery

In 1994, Nagamatsu and colleagues investigated the association between CPET-derived variables and outcome following upper gastrointestinal (GI) surgery. They analysed data from 52 patients who had a right thoracolaparotomy for thoracic oesophageal cancer, and observed significant differences in VO_{2max} and LT (both normalised to body surface area) between patients with and without postoperative cardiopulmonary complications. In a follow-up study, they retrospectively analysed data from 91 patients (mean age 59 years) who had undergone an oesophagectomy with three-field lymphadenectomy for squamous cell carcinoma and preoperative CPET.[42] Consistent with their original study, VO_{2max} values (normalised to body surface area) were significantly lower in the cohort of patients that experienced cardiopulmonary complications (789 mL/min/m^2) than in those without complications (966 mL/min/m^2) (p < 0.001). However, no association was observed between complications and LT. Further analysis revealed that VO_{2max} of 800 mL/min/m^2 was the optimal threshold to discriminate those at high risk of postoperative cardiopulmonary morbidity. Below this threshold, each 100 mL/min/m^2 decrease in VO_{2max} was accompanied by an increase in patient complication rate.

In a later study, Forshaw[43] investigated capacity of CPET markers to predict patients at increased risk of postoperative complications following oesophagectomy. The median age of patients within this study was 65 years (range 40–81 years). Consistent with previous CPET studies in patients undergoing upper GI surgery, the LT did not differ between those with and without cardiopulmonary complications. However, patients with postoperative cardiopulmonary complications had a significantly lower peak VO_2 (19.2 ± 5.1 mL/kg/min) than those without complications (21.4 ± 4.8 mL/kg/min) (p = 0.04). The association between peak VO_2 and postoperative cardiopulmonary complications was relatively weak (AUC, 0.63; 95% CI, 0.50–0.76).

The association between CPET variables and outcome following bariatric surgery was also investigated in 109 obese patients [mean body mass index (BMI) 48.1 kg/m^2] undergoing laparoscopic Roux-en-Y gastric bypass surgery.[29] Primary outcome variables assessed were death, unstable angina, myocardial infarction, deep vein thrombosis, pulmonary embolus, renal failure and stroke; secondary outcomes were hospital length of stay (LOS) and readmission. The population was divided into tertiles according to VO_2 peak values achieved during treadmill exercise. The rate of complications was significantly higher for the first tertile (n = 6, 16.2%) compared to the second and third tertiles (for both; n = 1, 2.8%) (p = 0.03). Similarly, hospital LOS was longer for the first tertile (3.8 days) than the second (2.9 days) and third tertiles (2.8 days) (p = 0.005). The threshold VO_2 peak value of 15.8 mL/kg/min, which was the upper boundary of the lowest tertile, had a sensitivity of 75% and a specificity of 73.3% to predict the occurrence of postoperative complications. These results indicate that for a morbidly obese population having bariatric surgery, a VO_2 peak less than or equal to 15.8 mL/kg/min has a reasonable capacity to predict those at increased risk of postoperative complications and longer hospital LOS.

Key Point

In upper gastrointestinal cancer surgery, peak VO_2 appears to be weakly associated with outcome, and the clinical utility of peak VO_2 or other CPET variables for prediction of postoperative outcome in this type of surgery is still uncertain.

Transplantation

In a study performed by Epstein and colleagues[44] in 2004, symptom-limited cardiopulmonary exercise testing conducted an average of approximately 15 months before surgery, was found to be associated with short-term outcome after hepatic transplantation. Specifically, they found that reduced aerobic capacity as defined by a reduced peak VO_2 (% predicted) and reduced VO_2 at LT (% of predicted peak VO_2), was associated with increased mortality during the first 100 days after hepatic transplantation. Non-survivors were more likely to have a peak VO_2 of less than 60% predicted (p = 0.04) and a VO_2 at LT less than 50% predicted (p = 0.03). This association persisted after controlling for duration and severity of liver disease, age, gender and time to transplantation; however, long-held reference values used for predicted variables were derived from small sample size populations and are deemed to be unreliable. Very recently, Snowden and colleagues[45] assessed the feasibility of preoperative submaximal CPET in determining the cardiopulmonary reserve in patients being assessed for liver transplantation and its potential for predicting 90-day post-transplant survival. One hundred eighty-two patients underwent CPET as part of their preoperative assessment for elective liver transplantation. One hundred sixty-five of the 182 patients (91%) successfully completed CPET. Sixty of the 182 patients (33%) underwent liver transplantation, and the mortality rate was 10% (6/60). The mean LT value was significantly higher for survivors versus non-survivors (12.0 ± 2.4 versus 8.4 ± 1.3 mL/min/kg, p < 0.001). Logistic regression revealed that LT, donor age, blood transfusions and fresh frozen plasma transfusions were significant univariate predictors of outcomes. In a multivariate analysis, only LT was retained as a significant predictor of mortality. A ROC curve analysis demonstrated sensitivity and specificity of 90.7% and 83.3%, respectively, with good model accuracy (CI 0.82–0.97, p = 0.001). The optimal LT level for survival was defined to be greater than 9 mL/min/kg. The predictive value was improved when the ideal weight was substituted for the actual body weight of a patient with refractory ascites, even after a correction for the donor's age.

DISCUSSION

This literature shows that CPET variables are reliably associated with outcome following major surgery. CPET also has utility in identifying the high-risk surgical patient. However, the optimal predictor of high risk appears to differ between surgery types, with LT shown to be the best indicator of higher-risk patients for major intra-abdominal surgery,[18,21,22,28] V_E/VCO_2 for AAA repair surgery,[30] and VO_2 peak for upper gastrointestinal and bariatric surgery.[29,42,43,46] However, it appears that the value of CPET is less clear in risk stratification before upper gastrointestinal and bariatric surgery. The evidence supporting preoperative CPET as a useful test to aid patient's and clinician's decisions in relation to surgical risk is, at present, incomplete. The literature comprises a number of small- and medium-sized studies on a limited range of surgical patients. A significant weakness in most of the included studies is the problem of "confounding by indication" due to lack of clinician blinding.[39] The effect of this will be to reduce the strength of association between predictor variable (CPET) and outcome, in relation to the true association. Variation in the type and strength of the association between CPET variable and outcome in different types of surgery is likely to be due to variation in the relative importance of different factors predisposing to adverse outcome; the relative contribution of surgical technique, perioperative care and patient physiological responses is likely to vary for different surgical procedures. For example, the consequences of anastomotic breakdown following oesophageal surgery may be more substantial than following lower gastrointestinal surgery. Furthermore, the current literature relating CPET variables to outcome is inconsistent in methods of analysis and presentation of data. This precludes firm conclusions with respect to choice of variable and optimal cut points for identifying high-risk patients for specific procedures.

One possibility is that CPET variables shown to be predictive of outcome in the literature are dependent on particular surgery types based on the individual stressors of certain operations.

In conclusion, for mixed intra-abdominal surgery, the ability of LT to predict all-cause mortality (AUC, 0.68)[22] was higher than that reported for the RCRI in a recent systematic review (AUC, 0.62).[47] Several studies have identified that CPET variables could be used in conjunction with other non-CPET markers [RCRI, visual sustained attention quotient (VSAQ), POSSUM] to enhance the capacity to predict perioperative risk.[21,30] This represents a potential opportunity to maximise our ability to identify high-risk patients before surgery; however adequately powered,

> **Key Point**
>
> Future studies should endeavour to use more robust study design (blinded studies with an appropriate sample size) and statistical methods that will properly evaluate the predictive capacity of CPET variables.

> **Key Points for Clinical Practice**
>
> 1. Risk prediction from CPET should always be evaluated in the context of the overall clinical picture.
>
> 2. Cardiopulmonary exercise testing can be used for risk stratification and perioperative patient management.
>
> 3. Specific CPET-derived variables seem to have particular predictive value for specific surgical types.
>
> 4. In general, a prudent approach, characterised by conservative estimation of perioperative risk, is likely to result in optimal patient outcomes, but this needs to be balanced against the increased resource usage (e.g. ICU bed days).
>
> 5. An LT of 11 mL/kg/min appears to be an acceptable threshold to use in a clinical setting to indicate increased perioperative risk following major intra-abdominal surgery, despite some indication that this value may lower in some centres.

prospective, blinded studies need to be conducted to clarify the role of CPET in preoperative risk prediction.

6. A V_E/VCO_2 greater than or equal to 42 should be used to help identify high-risk patients undergoing AAA repair surgery; however, hyperventilation should always be considered as this can artificially inflate this variable.

7. In upper gastrointestinal cancer surgery, peak VO_2 appears to be weakly associated with outcome, and the clinical utility of peak VO_2 or other CPET variables for prediction of postoperative outcome in this type of surgery is still uncertain.

8. Future studies should endeavour to use more robust study design (blinded studies with an appropriate sample size) and statistical methods that will properly evaluate the predictive capacity of CPET variables.

REFERENCES

1. Finan P, Greenaway K, Smith J, et al. (2011). National bowel cancer audit report [online]. Available from http://www.ic.nhs.uk/bowelreports [Accessed August, 2012].

2. Bayly PJ, Matthews JN, Dobson PM, et al. In-hospital mortality from abdominal aortic surgery in Great Britain and Ireland: Vascular Anaesthesia Society audit. Br J Surg. 2001;88(5):687-92.

3. NHS. (2012). National oesophago-gastric cancer audit [Online]. 2012. Available from http://www.ic.nhs.uk/services/national-clinical-audit-support-programme-ncasp/audit-reports/oesophago-gastric-cancer. [Accessed August, 2011].

4. Pearse RM, Harrison DA, James P, et al. Identification and characterisation of the high-risk surgical population in the United Kingdom. Crit Care. 2006;10(3):R81.

5. Barry MJ, Edgman-Levitan S. Shared decision making—pinnacle of patient-centered care. N Eng J Med. 2012;366(9):780-1.

6. Hightower CE, Riedel BJ, Feig BW, et al. A pilot study evaluating predictors of postoperative outcomes after major abdominal surgery: physiological capacity compared with the ASA physical status classification system. Br J Anaesth. 2010;104(4):465-71.

7. Menon KV, Farouk R. An analysis of the accuracy of P-POSSUM scoring for mortality risk assessment after surgery for colorectal cancer. Colorectal Dis. 2002;4(3):197-200.

8. Tekkis PP, Prytherch DR, Kocher HM, et al. Development of a dedicated risk-adjustment scoring system for colorectal surgery (colorectal POSSUM). Br J Surg. 2004;91(9):1174-82.

9. Edwards M, Whittle J, Ackland GL. Biomarkers to guide perioperative management. Postgrad Med J. 2011;87(1030):542-9.

10. Baron JF, Mundler O, Bertrand M, et al. Dipyridamole-thallium scintigraphy and gated radionuclide angiography to assess cardiac risk before abdmominal aortic surgery. N Engl J Med. 1994;330(10):663-9.

11. Shaw LJ, Eagle KA, Gersh BJ, et al. Meta-analysis of intravenous dipyridamole-thallium-201 imaging (1985 to 1994) and dobutamine echocardiography (1991 to 1994) for risk stratification before vascular surgery. J Am Coll Cardiol. 1996;27(4):787-98.

12. Halm EA, Browner WS, Tabau JF, et al. Echocardiography for assessing cardiac risk in patients having noncardiac surgery. Study of Perioperative Ischemia Research Group. Ann Intern Med. 1996;125(6):433-41.

13. Murray P, Whiting P, Hutchinson SP, et al. Preoperative shuttle walking testing and outcome after oesophagogastrectomy. Br J Anaesth. 2007;99(6):809-11.

14. Singh SJ, Morgan MD, Hardman AE. Comparison of oxygen uptake during a conventional treadmill test and the shuttle walking test in chronic airflow limitation. Eur Respir J. 1994;7:2016-20.

15. Struthers R, Erasmus P, Holmes K, et al. Assessing fitness for surgery: a comparison of questionnaire, incremental shuttle walk, and cardiopulmonary exercise testing in general surgical patients. Br J Anaesth. 2008;101(6):774-80.

16. Ross RM, Murthy JN, Wollak ID, et al. The six minute walk test accurately estimates mean peak oxygen uptake. BMC Pulm Med. 2010;10:31.

17. Guazzi M, Dickstein K, Vicenzi M, et al. Six-minute walk test and cardiopulmonary exercise testing in patients with chronic heart failure: a comparative analysis on clinical and prognostic insights. Circ Heart Fail. 2009;2(6):549-55.

18. Older P, Smith R, Hone R. Preoperative evaluation of cardiac failure and ischemia in elderly patients by cardiopulmonary exercise testing. Chest. 1993;104:701-4.

19. Simpson JC, Sutton H, Grocott MP. Cardiopulmonary exercise testing—a survey of current use in England. J Intensive Care Soc. 2009;10(4):275-8.

20. Ridgway ZA, Howell SJ. Cardiopulmonary exercise testing: a review of methods and applications in surgical patients. Eur J Anaesthesiol. 2010;27(10):858-65.

21. Snowden CP, Prentis JM, Anderson HL, et al. Submaximal cardiopulmonary exercise testing predicts complications and hospital length of stay in patients undergoing major elective surgery. Ann Surg. 2010;251(3):535-41.

22. Wilson RJ, Davies S, Yates D, et al. Impaired functional capacity is associated with all-cause mortality after major elective intra-abdominal surgery. Br J Anaesth. 2010;105(3):297-303.

23. Weisman IM, Marciniuk D, Martinez FJ, et al. ATS/ACCP statement on cardiopulmonary exercise testing. Am J Respir Crit Care Med. 2003;167(2):211-77.

24. Stringer W, Casaburi R, Older P. Cardiopulmonary exercise testing: does it improve perioperative care and outcome? Curr Opin Anaesthesiol. 2012;25(2):178-84.

25. Wasserman K, Hansen JE, Sue DY, et al. Principles of Exercise Testing and Interpretation: Pathophysiology and Clinical Applications. 4th Edition. Baltimore, Maryland: Lippincott Williams & Wilkins; 2005. p. 1-180.

26. Palange P, Ward SA, Carlsen KH, et al. Recommendations on the use of exercise testing in clinical practice. Eur Respir J. 2007;29(1):185-209.

27. Fleisher LA, Beckman JA, Brown KA, et al. ACC/AHA 2007 guidelines on perioperative cardiovascular evaluation and care for noncardiac surgery: a report of the American College of Cardiology/American Heart Association Task Force on Practice Guidelines (Writing Committee to Revise the 2002 Guidelines on Perioperative Cardiovascular Evaluation for Noncardiac Surgery): developed in collaboration with the American Society of Echocardiography, American Society of Nuclear Cardiology, Heart Rhythm Society, Society of Cardiovascular Anesthesiologists, Society for Cardiovascular Angiography and Interventions, Society for Vascular Medicine and Biology, and Society for Vascular Surgery. Circulation. 2007;116(17):e418-99.

28. Older P, Hall A, Hader R. Cardiopulmonary exercise testing as a screening test for perioperative management of major surgery in the elderly. Chest. 1999;116(2):355-62.

29. McCullough PA, Gallagher MJ, Dejong AT, et al. Cardiorespiratory fitness and short-term complications after bariatric surgery. Chest. 2006;130(2):517-25.

30. Carlisle J, Swart M. Mid-term survival after abdominal aortic aneurysm surgery predicted by cardiopulmonary exercise testing. Br J Surg. 2007;94(8):966-9.

31. West M, Jack S, Grocott MP. Perioperative cardiopulmonary exercise testing in the elderly. Best Prac Res Clin Anaesthesiol. 2011;25(3):427-37.

32. Smith TB, Stonell C, Purkayastha S, et al. Cardiopulmonary exercise testing as a risk assessment method in non-cardiopulmonary surgery: a systematic review. Anaesthesia. 2009;64(8):883-93.

33. Hennis PJ, Meale PM, Grocott MP. Cardiopulmonary exercise testing for the evaluation of perioperative risk in non-cardiopulmonary surgery. Postgrad Med J. 2011;87(1030):550-7.

34. Beaver WL, Wasserman K, Whipp J. A new method for detecting anaerobic threshold by gas exchange. J Appl Physiol. 1986;60(6):2020-7.

35. Sue DY, Wasserman K, Moricca RB, et al. Metabolic acidosis during exercise in patients with chronic obstructive pulmonary disease. Use of the V-slope method for anaerobic threshold determination. Chest. 1988;94(5):931-8.

36. Hopker JG, Jobson SA, Pandit JJ. Controversies in the physiological basis of the 'anaerobic threshold' and their implications for clinical cardiopulmonary exercise testing. Anaesthesia. 2011;66(2):111-23.

37. Sinclair RC, Danjoux GR, Goodridge V, et al. Determination of the anaerobic threshold in the pre-operative assessment clinic: inter-observer measurement error. Anaesthesia. 2009 Nov;64(11):1192-5.

38. Older P, Hall A. Clinical review: how to identify high-risk surgical patients. Crit Care. 2004;8(5):369-72.

39. Grocott MP, Pearse RM. Prognostic studies of perioperative risk: robust methodology is needed. Br J Anaesth. 2010;105(3):243-5.

40. Junejo MA, Mason JM. Cardiopulmonary exercise testing for preoperative risk assessment before hepatic resection. Br J Surg. 2012;99(8):1097-104.

41. Nugent AM, Riley M, Megarry J, et al. Cardiopulmonary exercise testing in the pre-operative assessment of patients for repair of abdominal aortic aneurysm. Ir J Med Sci. 1998;167(4):238-41.

42. Nagamatsu Y, Shima I, Yamana H, et al. Preoperative evaluation of cardiopulmonary reserve with the use of expired gas analysis during exercise testing in patients with squamous cell carcinoma of the thoracic esophagus. J Thorac Cardiovasc Surg. 2001;121(6):1064-8.

43. Forshaw MJ, Strauss DC, Davies AR, et al. Is cardiopulmonary exercise testing a useful test before esophagectomy? Ann Thorac Surg. 2008;85(1):294-9.

44. Epstein SK, Freeman RB, Khayat A, et al. Aerobic capacity is associated with 100-day outcome after hepatic transplantation. Liver transplantation: official publication of the American Association for the Study of Liver Diseases and the International Liver Transplantation Society. Liver Transpl. 2004;10(3):418-24.

45. Snowden CP, Anderson H. Preoperative optimization: rationale and process: is it economic sense? Curr Opin Anaesthesiol. 2012;25(2):210-6.

46. Forshaw MJ, Strauss DC, Davies AR, et al. Reply. Ann Thorac Surg. 2009;87(2):671-2.

47. Ford MK, Beattie WS, Wijeysundera DN. Systematic review: prediction of perioperative cardiac complications and mortality by the revised cardiac risk index. Ann Intern Med. 2010;152(7):26-35.

4

Breast Reconstruction: How do we Measure and Define Patient's Quality of Life and Satisfaction?

Anushka Chaudhry, Zoë Ellen Winters

INTRODUCTION

In the United Kingdom, 30–40% of the 44,000 women diagnosed annually with breast cancer will undergo mastectomy.[1] The UK National Mastectomy and Breast Reconstruction Audit (NMBRA) surveyed 18,000 women between 2008 and 2009, and although nearly half of women were offered the option of immediate reconstruction,[1] approximately 3,000 underwent immediate breast reconstruction compared to delayed reconstructions in 2,000 women.[1] In 2002, the National Institute of Clinical Excellence (NICE) issued guidelines stating that all women should be offered immediate breast reconstruction following mastectomy.[2] At that time, only 7% of women underwent an immediate breast reconstruction.[3] The current rate of immediate procedures has risen to 21%, but with a large variation of 9–43% across the UK National Health Service (NHS), reflecting a wide variation in practice.[1,3] The NICE issued a further statement in 2009 pertaining to breast reconstruction that health care professionals should discuss reconstruction with every woman recommended for mastectomy, and that women should be made aware of all the possible reconstructive options.[2] This approach is subject to relevant considerations such as co-morbidities and the need for adjuvant therapy, particularly post-mastectomy radiotherapy (PMRT).[4-6]

> **Key Point**
>
> NMBRA has provided an important benchmark for measuring standard of care and patient satisfaction in the UK.

TYPES OF RECONSTRUCTION

There are four main breast reconstructive options available following mastectomy.[6] These can be performed immediately at the time of the mastectomy or as a second delayed procedure at varying intervals after mastectomy. Most commonly performed in the UK is an immediate implant only breast reconstruction (37%).[1,6] The use of a microvascular 'free' flap is most frequently used in 33% of delayed breast reconstruction procedures.[1,6] The available reconstruction options are (Table 4.1):

1. Insertion of an expander or fixed-volume implant, which is usually a two-stage procedure involving insertion of a first-stage expander implant into a submuscular pocket of pectoralis major and serratus anterior chest wall muscles during mastectomy. The tissue expander implant is inflated intraoperatively with saline and as an outpatient over 1 month. Implant expansion is followed by adjuvant chemotherapy and/or PMRT. Completion of the latter treatments is followed by the second surgical replacement of the expander by a permanent implant alone or a delayed tissue-based flap reconstruction of the breast.[6]
2. Implant-assisted flap reconstruction is the insertion of an expander or implant accompanied by tissue from either the patient's back or abdomen.[6]
3. Autologous tissue only pedicled flap utilises the intact vascular pedicle to supply the flap derived most commonly from the abdomen called the transverse rectus abdominis myocutaneous (TRAM) flap comprising abdominal skin, fat and rectus muscle. The other commonly performed type uses a vascular pedicled flap of back skin, fat and latissimus dorsi (LD) muscle and is known as the extended autologous LD (ALD). Both procedures utilise donor site (abdomen or back) tissues such as LD muscle, fat and skin, referred to as muscle sacrificing.[6]
4. Autologous tissue only 'free' flap utilises the microvascular dissection, transection and distant micro re-anastomosis to a donor site blood vessel. The commonest microvascular type flaps are the 'free' TRAM and deep inferior epigastric perforator (DIEP) reconstructions comprising abdominal skin and fat. Other 'free' flaps such as superior gluteal artery perforators (SGAP) and inferior gluteal artery perforators (IGAP) that utilise gluteal/buttock tissues may also be used.[6]

TABLE 4.1: Data from the NMBRA, illustrating the proportion of immediate and delayed reconstructions in the UK

Types and timings of breast reconstruction				
Type of surgery	Immediate reconstruction	%	Delayed reconstruction	%
Implant/expander-only	1,246	36.8	281	16.2
Pedicle flap + implant/expander	735	21.7	438	25.3
Pedicle flap (autologous)	932	27.5	446	25.8
Free flap	476	14.0	566	32.7
Total	3,389		1,731	

WHAT DO WE MEAN BY 'PATIENT SATISFACTION?' PATIENT REPORTED OUTCOME MEASURES

Clinical outcomes such as mortality and complication rates are important, but there is increasing awareness and evidence of the significance of assessing patient self-reported outcomes when evaluating the effects of reconstructive surgery over time.[7,8] Patient reported outcome measures (PROMs) are measures of a patient's health status or health-related quality of life (HRQL) as well as satisfaction.[7,8] The concept of HRQL and its determinants has evolved since 1980s to encompass those aspects of overall quality of life that can be clearly shown to affect health, comprising either physical or mental issues, including functioning (role, social), sexual issues, satisfaction with outcomes and body image.[9,10] They are typically short, self-reported questionnaires measuring the patients' HRQL at a single point in time.[7] The information from PROMs before and after an intervention provides an overarching and comprehensive assessment of the surgical outcomes and quality of care.[7] Patient reported outcomes (PROs) supplement clinical evaluations by providing the patients' perceptions of the disease and treatment and have contributed towards formulating NICE guidelines as well as providing key outcomes in the NMBRA that serve as a national benchmark.[1]

Studies comparing specific types of breast reconstruction demonstrate that patients have differing views from clinicians when self-reporting their outcomes. This divergence of opinion endorses the combined assessments of PROMs as well as standardised clinical outcomes.[5] Historically, most studies evaluating breast reconstruction practice have focused on clinician-reported outcomes, such as surgical complications that may or may not be relevant to patients.[11] It is difficult to derive sound evidence from systematic reviews on HRQL as a primary outcome after all types of breast reconstruction.[12,13] Studies to date have been methodologically poorly designed and underpowered with limited follow-up.[12,13] There are virtually no randomised trials (n = 2) and few prospective longitudinal studies (n = 11), with the majority of studies being retrospective in design.[12,13] Furthermore, many studies use PROMs that are generic for cancer in general as well as breast cancer that may be complementary to those questionnaires developed specifically to assess HRQL after types of breast reconstruction.[12-14]

> **Key Point**
> PROMs are measures of a patient's health status or HRQL as well as satisfaction.

Measuring Patient Reported Outcome Measures

Generic methods of measuring patient satisfaction have formed the basis of much of the evidence used to date when discussing breast reconstruction.[15] The short form (SF)-36 is a multipurpose questionnaire that is used to assess functional health and well-being scores covering physical and mental issues.[16] European and American cancer patients and health care professionals have been studied to develop and validate PROMs that assess all aspects of general HRQL in cancer and breast cancer. The European Organization for the Research and Treatment of Cancer (EORTC) has developed the general cancer questionnaire called the QLQ-C30 and a supplementary questionnaire used to assess patients with breast cancer, the QLQ-BR23.[17] The Functional Assessment of Cancer Therapy (FACT) questionnaires have been developed for general cancer (FACT-G) and breast cancer patients (FACT-B) and are complementary in the assessments of patients' HRQL.[18] The Hopwood Body Image Scale (BIS)[19] has also been extensively used, with all these PROMs having high reliability and validity. However, more recently measures of satisfaction have been specifically developed.[20] The Michigan Breast Reconstruction and Outcomes Study (MBROS) developed a validated questionnaire assessing patient satisfaction in general (MBROS-S), as well as with aesthetic results relating to body image (MBROS-BI) after breast reconstruction.[14]

> **Key Point**
>
> PROMs most commonly used in the field are the BREAST-Q, EORTC (QLQ-C30 and BR23), FACT-G, FACT-B and SF-36.

BREAST-Q

The development of the BREAST-Q was published in 2009 and was validated in three breast reconstruction specific procedures (augmentation, breast reduction and reconstruction).[20] The aim of the BREAST-Q was to represent the whole patient experience. The instrument was developed by interviewing patients from five centres in the United States and Canada. Figure 4.1 demonstrates the six resulting scales or domains comprising individual items/questions that covered HRQL and patient satisfaction.[20]

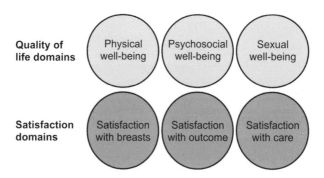

Figure 4.1: The BREAST-Q conceptual framework

These independent scales examine the issues most important to women undergoing each breast procedure. By developing the scales/domains and items/questions specific to each surgical group, each questionnaire has the potential to be more sensitive to those patients' perceptions. This allows information relating to the various HRQL domains to be individually assessed in different clinical scenarios. An important example is the quality of care for patients undergoing mastectomy with or without breast reconstruction of which the core elements include:[1,14]

- Involvement in decisions
- Provision of appropriate information
- Provision of appropriate choices and access to care
- Satisfaction with the behaviour of doctors and nurses
- Pain control
- Treatment with respect and dignity throughout the episode.

Therefore, if a patient is satisfied with the overall result, but not a specific aspect of her care, such as the provision of information, the BREAST-Q provides this information. Such an approach endorses the value of assessing PROMs.

MANAGING EXPECTATIONS

The primary goal of reconstruction is to improve a woman's body image and to fulfil her expectations regarding the appearance of her breasts following surgery.[6] Recognising expectations is becoming more difficult due to the trend towards speedier systems of care. Decisions regarding breast reconstruction are now usually made soon after the diagnosis of breast cancer. At this highly emotional and stressful time, women make rapid, highly intuitive decisions when confronted by the threat of breast cancer. Primarily, issues of survival are prioritised around the time of diagnosis.[21] It must be made clear to women that breast reconstruction has not been shown to affect the incidence of or the detection of local recurrence.[21] In research of other surgical areas, patient dissatisfaction was closely related to failure to meet patient expectations (superseding the technical success of the procedure).[22] For example in cardiac surgery, positive expectations for health after heart transplantation have been associated with better postoperative scores for mood, adjustment to illness and HRQL, even in patients who encountered health setbacks.[23] Similarly, in patients who underwent surgery for sciatica, those with favourable expectations about surgery had better outcomes than those with less favourable expectations.[24] This was also seen in urology patients undergoing transurethral resection of the prostate, with positive expectations leading to improved reports of health at 3 months after surgery.[25] Furthermore, in other areas of healthcare, patient expectation has been closely related to satisfaction and HRQL.[22] In primary care, higher patient satisfaction with care and compliance with treatment have been demonstrated in those with realistic expectations of their health. Health care professionals must address patient expectations in order to recognise those that are 'unrealistic'.[22] On this basis, health care professionals should endeavour to improve patient knowledge and education through giving adequate information as in evidence-based informed consent.[12,13,26] In breast reconstruction, where there may be more than one surgical option that is technically feasible, current recommendations are that the choice of procedure should include a standardised informed consent and exploration of patients' preferences including their attitudes to illness and risk within the context of the clinical evidence.[12,13,22] Such an approach may enhance shared decision making and be a way of managing patients' expectations.[22] Shared decision-making 'reconceptualises' the roles and responsibilities of patients and health care professionals in improving health.[27] In a large cohort study of membership candidates from the Royal College of General Practitioners (MRCGP), their five 'best' recorded consultations were assessed to determine their ability to elicit patients' ideas, concerns and expectations.[28] The study results showed that after 3 years of postgraduate training, doctors in general practice showed only limited ability to elicit PROs. A national patient survey showed that 1 in 3 patients in primary care and 1 in 2 hospital patients would have liked greater involvement in decisions about their care (Department of Health, 2007).[29] Fundamentally, the ability to share decisions with patients must be seen as a core component of professionalism, where doctors support patients to make decisions rather than demonstrating their expertise.[30]

> **Key Point**
>
> Patients' preferences should be explored along with attitudes to risk and illness when obtaining informed consent for breast reconstruction.

DECISION MAKING: 'NOTHING ABOUT ME WITHOUT ME'

In 2010, the NHS constitution health reforms encouraged patients to participate in appropriate treatment or management options on the basis of the best available evidence.[1,12,13,21] A high quality decision about breast reconstruction requires that patients:

1. Should have knowledge about reconstruction (including risks and benefits).
2. Should receive treatment that is consistent with preferences and goals
3. Are involved in making decisions about their care.

In the UK, patient satisfaction with overall experience, clinician and care received was generally high. In order to optimise the consent process, however, health care professionals must use evidence that integrates both sound PROMs methodology and give accurate reporting of complications.[1,12,13,21] In two systematic reviews, fewer than 20% of studies predefined the reported complications and less than half failed to mention risk factors for adverse outcomes.[31] This is a concern as there is a significant underestimation of the contribution of complications to HRQL and patient satisfaction.[1] The key findings of the NMBRA pertaining to complications will provide a benchmark for improvement and may enhance the informed consenting process.[1]

> **Key Point**
>
> Complication reporting is poor in the literature. Based on key findings from the NMBRA and other studies, clinicians should strive to document accurately their personal complications in order to optimise the consent process.

KEY FINDINGS OF THE NMBRA FOURTH REPORT

The fourth report of the NMBRA provides information on clinician-reported data such as patient characteristics, treatments received and complications both early and late.[1] It elaborates on patient-reported data about the experience of care and quality of life outcomes using the BREAST-Q.[1] Key findings reported are on:

1. **Pain:** Pain is experienced as severe within the first 24 hours after 16.5% of immediate reconstructions and following 20.1% of delayed procedures. This alarming rate significantly exceeds recommendations from the Audit Commission (1997) in which this complication should be experienced in less than 5% of patients.[1] The trends in severe pain are shown in Table 4.2.

TABLE 4.2: Pain experienced from time of surgery to 18 months reported in the NMBRA

Operation	Severe pain (%)		Continuing pain (%)	
	First 24 hours	*First week*	*3 months*	*18 months*
Mastectomy	6.2	5.2	49	7–12
Immediate reconstruction	16.5	11.4	51.9	4–8
Delayed reconstruction	20.1	9.4	40.9	1–9

2. **Early and late complications:** One in ten women had a complication within the first 30 days after surgery (Table 4.3) with a relatively high rate of infection requiring antibiotics and high rates of re-admission for unplanned treatment or surgery.

TABLE 4.3: Complications at 3 months after surgery for types of breast reconstruction from the NMBRA

Complication	Mastectomy (%)	Immediate (%)	Delayed (%)
Re-admission for unplanned treatment or surgery	8.9	15.8	13.9
Bleeding requiring transfusion or surgery	1.1	1.7	1.9
Infection requiring antibiotics	17.0	24.1	26.8
Implant loss	N/A	8.9	6.9
Flap loss	Total	N/A	< 1
	Partial		5

Abbreviation: *N/A: Not applicable*

Few studies in the systematic reviews analyse the effects of either early or long-term complications on women' HRQL after breast reconstructions.[12,13] The present author has shown the significant adverse effects of early complications (within 3 months) affecting virtually all aspects of a woman's HRQL upto 12 months after surgery.[32] This impacts on global feelings of well-being, functioning, fatigue, pain, worse breast symptoms and greater depression.[32] Complications occurring after 3 months upto 1 year cause persistent breast symptoms and worse body image.[32]

3. **Mental issues and psychological support:** In the NMBRA, the proportion of women who reported receiving psychological support or counselling upto 18 months after their surgery was 30.3% for mastectomy-only patients, 27.6% for immediate reconstruction patients and 16.9% for delayed reconstruction patients.[1] Relatively few women received psychological support from a health care professional within the 3-month postoperative period. This may be partially due to limited access to psychosocial support in some units and also a tendency towards early hospital discharge, leaving minimal time for the breast care nurse to see the patient postoperatively. The NICE guidelines (2002) for breast cancer state that 'Psychosocial support should be available at every stage to help patients and their families cope with the effects of the disease'.[1,21]

The NMBRA assessed emotional well-being using various domains from the BREAST-Q such as overall well-being, attractiveness and confidence in the social setting. The results showed upward trends in the levels of emotional satisfaction in patients undergoing immediate and delayed breast reconstructions compared to mastectomy alone as shown in Table 4.4.

TABLE 4.4: Emotional well-being at 18 months recorded in the NMBRA[1]

Operation	Range of emotional well-being scores (%)
Mastectomy	45–77
Immediate	61–85
Delayed	69–92

4. **Satisfaction outcomes:** Breast reconstruction patients reported higher levels of satisfaction with appearance, confidence in a social setting and satisfaction with their sex life compared to those who underwent mastectomy alone. Satisfaction was slightly higher after delayed reconstruction of the breast compared to immediate procedures. It can be difficult to compare satisfaction outcomes of patients undergoing immediate versus delayed reconstructions due to the fact that the latter group have lived without a breast for a period of time. It may be considered that such women have had longer to deal with the loss of a breast with its associated 'grieving' so to speak, thus modifying their expectations of a subsequent breast reconstruction with possibly higher levels of satisfaction. In Table 4.5, combined scores are shown for 'satisfied' and 'very satisfied' on an item-level satisfaction scoring

system (% of 'satisfied' and 'very satisfied') for the HRQL domains after breast reconstruction in the NMBRA.

TABLE 4.5: Mean outcome scores for satisfaction at 18 months postoperatively. Scores were adjusted for women's age, deprivation index, performance status, smoking status, and whether they had undergone radiotherapy and/or chemotherapy postoperatively

Operation		Breast area appearance (%)	Emotional well-being (%)	Physical well-being (%)	Sexual well-being (%)
Mastectomy only		56	63	73	39
Immediate	Implant only	54	65	74	44
	Pedicle with implant	63	72	75	50
	Autologous free flap	64	70	73	49
	Free flap	63	70	75	49
Delayed	Implant only	57	66	76	49
	Pedicle with implant	68	76	76	58
	Autologous free flap	69	74	77	56
	Free flap	73	78	80	63

5. **Satisfaction and body image:** Body image is defined as the mental picture of one's body, an attitude about the physical self, appearance, general health, feelings of 'wholeness', normal functioning and sexuality. All women diagnosed with breast cancer, regardless of ethnicity, have concerns regarding sexuality and body image.[19,33] This has been described in young women undergoing surgery for breast cancer. It is not surprising, therefore, that assessment of body image impacts greatly on patient satisfaction and PROMs. Studies have found that women who contemplated breast reconstruction before mastectomy were the least satisfied with their preoperative body image.[19] This may indicate a possible reason for seeking reconstruction. Table 4.6 shows outcomes of patient satisfaction relating to body image for immediate and delayed breast reconstructions. The overall satisfaction, satisfaction with abdominal appearance and with rippling of implant are combined score percentages of 'satisfied' and 'very satisfied'. Satisfaction with the donor site, pain/stiffness and abdominal functional impairment are percentage scores of whether women were bothered 'most' or 'all of the time'. Of note, there is no significant difference in patients' feeling of pain or symptoms of back stiffness between the implant with flap groups and the autologous reconstructions in immediate and delayed procedures.[1]

TABLE 4.6: Satisfaction outcomes range of scores as a percentage, relating to body image for breast reconstructions in the NMBRA

	Immediate (%)				Delayed (%)			
	Implant only	Implant with flap	Autologous LD	TRAM /DIEP	Implant only	Implant with flap	Autologous LD	TRAM /DIEP
Overall satisfaction	59–90				72–93			
Bothered with donor site (LD)	N/A	6–14	8–15	N/A	N/A	4–12	7–16	N/A
Pain/ stiffness		7–21	8–25			5–23	5–22	
Abdominal functional impairment	N/A			6–13	N/A			2–11
Satisfied with abdominal appearance	N/A			71–84	N/A			76–88
Satisfaction with rippling of implant	71–72	82–84	N/A		85–87	86–90	N/A	

Abbreviations: LD: Latissimus dorsi; TRAM: Transverse rectus abdominis myocutaneous; DIEP: Deep inferior epigastric perforator; N/A: Not applicable

ADJUVANT TREATMENTS AND EFFECTS ON HRQL AFTER BREAST RECONSTRUCTION

There is very little international data on the effects of PMRT after types of breast reconstruction and how this may affect HRQL.[12,13] Despite well-known adverse cosmetic sequelae of radiation on implant-based breast reconstructions, women may retain satisfaction with their reconstructed breasts which is evident over 5 years using a cross-sectional analysis of women undergoing different types of LD breast reconstruction.[5,13] Furthermore, the NMBR audit does not analyse the impact of PMRT on patients' satisfaction within any of the types of breast reconstructions studied.[1] In a large prospective longitudinal cohort, using a range of predefined HRQL domains from EORTC C30, BR23, FACT-B, BIS, anxiety and depression, there are no effects of PMRT on any of the areas of quality of life examined, such as global HRQL, functioning, fatigue, pain, breast and arm symptoms over 12 months.[32] By contrast, chemotherapy significantly adversely affected nearly all HRQL domains (except arm symptoms) over a 12-month period.[32] None of the four prospective studies in two systematic reviews evaluated the numbers of women who received chemotherapy and did not account for its potential effects on HRQL after breast reconstruction.[12,13] We have shown that it is important to consider the longer-term effects of chemotherapy on HRQL in women undergoing breast reconstruction as part of their informed consent.[32] This is also not an area reported on in the NMBR audit.[1] There is, therefore, a need for further work to be done in terms of evaluating how the effects of adjuvant treatments may influence patient satisfaction.

> **Key Point**
>
> Further work is required to investigate the findings in the NMBRA to establish even better evidence as to the effects of these surgeries on patients' HRQL.

CONCLUSIONS

The findings from the UK NMBR audit begin to address specific areas relating to patient satisfaction following different types and timings of breast reconstruction over 18 months.[1] The next step needs to build on this work by further analysing these issues over time but at the same time allowing for the integration of key determinants that are known to influence HRQL such as age, socio-demographic differences, ethnicity, surgical complications and adjuvant treatments.[32] Only then can we start to get a more discriminatory view of the burgeoning 'truth' or evidence of true clinical outcomes that pertain to both patient self-reported outcomes as well as traditional clinician assessments.

> **Key Points**
>
> 1. The NMBRA has provided an important benchmark for measuring standard of care and patient satisfaction in the UK.
> 2. PROMs are measures of a patient's health status or HRQL as well as satisfaction.
> 3. PROMS most commonly used in the field are the BREAST-Q, EORTC (QLQ-C30 and BR23), FACT-G and FACT-B, and SF-36.
> 4. Patients' preferences should be explored along with attitudes to risk and illness when obtaining informed consent for breast reconstruction.
> 5. Complication reporting is poor in the literature. Based on key findings from the NMBRA and other studies, clinicians should strive to document accurately their individual complications in order to optimise the consent process.
> 6. Further work is required to investigate the findings in the NMBRA to establish even better evidence as to the effects of these surgeries on patients' HRQL.

ACKNOWLEDGEMENTS

We would like to thank Ms Grania Pickard and Vali Balta for the preparation of this chapter as well as all the patients whose kind participation in the group's invited trials has enabled the advancement of clinical evidence in the field.

REFERENCES

1. NHS The Information Centre. (2009). Masectomy and breast reconstruction audit. [online] Available from: http://www.ic.nhs.uk/mbr. [Accessed August, 2012].
2. Mayor S. NICE updates guidance on medical and surgical treatment for early and advanced breast cancer. BMJ. 2009;7693:2.
3. Jeevan R, Cromwell DA, Browne JP, et al. Regional variation in use of immediate breast reconstruction after mastectomy for breast cancer in England. Eur J Surg Oncol. 2010;36(8):750-5.

4. Javaid M, Song F, Leinster S, et al. Radiation effects on the cosmetic outcomes of immediate and delayed autologous breast reconstruction: an argument about timing. J Plast Reconstr Aesthet Surg. 2006;59(1):16-26.

5. Thomson HJ, Potter S, Greenwood RJ, et al. A prospective longitudinal study of cosmetic outcome in immediate latissimus dorsi breast reconstruction and the influence of radiotherapy. Ann Surg Oncol. 2008;15(4):1081-91.

6. Cordeiro PG. Breast reconstruction after surgery for breast cancer. N Engl J Med. 2008;359(15):1590-601.

7. Devlin AJ, Appleby J. (2010). Getting the most out of PROMS. Putting health outcomes at the heart of NHS decision-making. The King's Fund. [Online] Available from: http://www.kingsfund.org.uk/publications. [Accessed August, 2012].

8. Cano SJ, Klassen A, Pusic AL. The science behind quality-of-life measurement: a primer for plastic surgeons. Plast Reconstr Surg. 2009;123(3):98e-106e.

9. Rowland JH, Hewitt M, Ganz PA. Cancer survivorship: a new challenge in delivering quality cancer care. J Clin Oncol. 2006;24(32):5101-4.

10. Goodwin PJ, Black JT, Bordeleau LJ, et al. Health-related quality-of-life measurement in randomized clinical trials in breast cancer--taking stock. J Natl Cancer Inst. 2003;95(4):263-81.

11. Morrow M, Pusic AL. Time for a new era in outcomes reporting for breast reconstruction. J Natl Cancer Inst. 2011;103(1):5-7.

12. Winters ZE, Benson JR, Pusic AL. A systematic review of the clinical evidence to guide treatment recommendations in breast reconstruction based on patient-reported outcome measures and health-related quality of life. Ann Surg. 2010;252(6):929-42.

13. Lee C, Sunu C, Pignone M. Patient-reported outcomes of breast reconstruction after mastectomy: a systematic review. J Am Coll Surg. 2009;209(1):123-33.

14. Pusic AL, Chen CM, Cano S, et al. Measuring quality of life in cosmetic and reconstructive breast surgery: a systematic review of patient-reported outcomes instruments. Plast Reconstr Surg. 2007;120(4):823-37; discussion 38-9.

15. Garratt A, Schmidt L, Mackintosh A, et al. Quality of life measurement: bibliographic study of patient assessed health outcome measures. BMJ. 2002;324(7351):1417.

16. John E. Ware Jr. (Australian Health Outcomes Collaboration) (2005). SF-36® Health Survey (Version 1.0). University of Wollongong. Available from: http://ahsri.uow.edu.au/ahoc/documents/sf36review.pdf. [Accessed August 2012].

17. Sprangers MA, Groenvold M, Arraras JI, et al. The European Organization for Research and Treatment of Cancer breast cancer-specific quality-of-life questionnaire module: first results from a three-country field study. J Clin Oncol. 1996;14(10):2756-68.

18. Brady MJ, Cella DF, Mo F, et al. Reliability and validity of the Functional Assessment of Cancer Therapy-Breast quality-of-life instrument. J Clin Oncol. 1997;15(3):974-86.

19. Hopwood P, Fletcher I, Lee A, et al. A body image scale for use with cancer patients. Eur J Cancer. 2001;37(2):189-97.

20. Pusic AL, Klassen AF, Scott AM, et al. Development of a new patient-reported outcome measure for breast surgery: the BREAST-Q. Plast Reconstr Surg. 2009;124(2):345-53.

21. Association of Breast Surgery at Baso 2009. Surgical guidelines for the management of breast cancer. Eur J Surg Oncol. 2009;35 Suppl 1:1-22.

22. Pusic AL, Klassen AF, Snell L, et al. Measuring and managing patient expectations for breast reconstruction: impact on quality of life and patient satisfaction. Expert Rev Pharmacoecon Outcomes Res. 2012;12(2):149-58.

23. Leedham B, Meyerowitz BE, Muirhead J, et al. Positive expectations predict health after heart transplantation. Health Psychol. 1995;14(1):74-9.

24. Lutz GK, Butzlaff ME, Atlas SJ, et al. The relation between expectations and outcomes in surgery for sciatica. J Gen Int Med. 1999;14(12):740-4.

25. Marschall-Kehrel D, Roberts RG, Brubaker L. Patient-reported outcomes in overactive bladder: the influence of perception of condition and expectation for treatment benefit. Urology. 2006;68(2 Suppl):29-37.

26. Guerra CE, McDonald VJ, Ravenell KL, et al. Effect of race on patient expectations regarding their primary care physicians. Fam Pract. 2008;25(1):49-55.

27. Marshall M, Bibby J. Supporting patients to make the best decisions. BMJ. 2011;342. d2117.

28. Campion P, Foulkes J, Neighbour R, et al. Patient centredness in the MRCGP video examination: analysis of large cohort. Membership of the Royal College of General Practitioners. BMJ. 2002;325(7366):691-2.

29. Department of Health. (2007). Report on the National Patient Choice Survey, England - July 2007. [Online]. Available from http://www.dh.gov.uk/en/Publication-sandstatistics/Publications/PublicationsStatistics/DH_081108. [Accessed Auugust 2012].

30. Stanton E, Lemer C, Marshall M. An evolution of professionalism. J R Soc Med. 2011;104(2):48-9.

31. Potter S, Brigic A, Whiting PF, et al. Reporting clinical outcomes of breast reconstruction: a systematic review. J Natl Cancer Inst. 2011;103(1):31-46.

32. Winters ZE, Haviland J, Reece-Smith A, et al. A multicentre prospective cohort study evaluating health related quality of life after types of immediate latissimus dorsi (LD) breast reconstruction. Cancer Research Suppl. 2011;71(24):318s.

33. Manganiello A, Hoga LA, Reberte LM, et al. Sexuality and quality of life of breast cancer patients post mastectomy. Eur J Oncol Nurs. 2011;15(2):167-72.

5 | Surgery for Benign Breast Conditions

Christina Summerhayes, Avi Agrawal, Rachel Oeppen,
Ramsey I Cutress

INTRODUCTION

The majority of patients presenting to a symptomatic breast clinic do not have breast cancer. In many cases, reassurance alone is sufficient; however there are a range of benign breast conditions that may pose a diagnostic challenge or prove difficult to manage. It is important to distinguish between benign 'disease', which implies abnormality, and aberrations of normal development and involution (ANDI). This chapter describes recent changes that have occurred in both diagnosis and management of gynaecomastia, mastalgia, nipple discharge, breast sepsis and benign lesions. These are selected as topics because they are frequently encountered in the breast clinic, and because there have been recent changes and developments in their management. In some cases, these will constitute ANDI rather than 'disease'.

GYNAECOMASTIA

Gynaecomastia is the benign enlargement of male breast tissue. It is characterised histologically by hyperplasia of the stromal and ductal tissue, and should be distinguished from pseudogynaecomastia, which is caused by excess in fat without change in the stromal or ductal tissue. Presentation can occur at any age with up to a third of men affected at some point during their life. The incidence of gynaecomastia peaks during adolescence when it is very common and usually self-limiting,[1] and increases again with age in the later decades of life.

It is postulated that gynaecomastia is caused by imbalances between oestrogen and androgen levels or altered responsiveness of the breast to these hormones. The causes may be physiological, pathological, drug induced or idiopathic, and taking a careful medical history, including use of recreational and performance-enhancing drugs is important. Secondary causes are less common, but are well described and include Klinefelter's syndrome, testicular feminisation, hermaphroditism, adrenal carcinoma, hepatic disease, primary and secondary hypogonadism, testicular tumours, hyperthyroidism, renal disease and malnutrition.[2] Clinical examination may demonstrate evidence of secondary causes. The degree of gynaecomastia is categorised (Simon's classification)[3] into three groups depending on parenchymal volume enlargement and skin excess (Table 5.1), and although 80% of male patients attending a breast unit with a breast lump are ultimately diagnosed with gynaecomastia, breast cancer should be excluded (Fig. 5.1).[4] Breast cancer is usually eccentric within the breast and unilateral, whereas gynaecomastia is usually concentric, subareolar and bilateral.

TABLE 5.1: Gynaecomastia—Simon grading[3]

Grade	Clinical appearance
I	Small but visible breast development with little redundant skin
IIa	Moderate breast development with no redundant skin
IIb	Moderate breast development with redundant skin
III	Marked breast development with much redundant skin

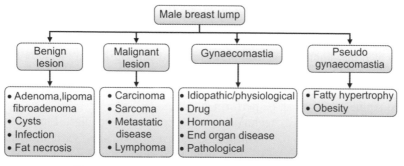

Figure 5.1: Differential diagnosis of a male breast lump

Investigations

Investigations are performed to exclude breast cancer or other pathological causes if clinically indicated, and algorithms for investigation have been developed.[4] The imaging modality chosen for primary investigation varies by institution but there is evidence that mammography is more sensitive than ultrasonography (95% vs 89%), although specificity for both approaches is 95%.[5] If breast cancer is suspected, core needle biopsy is recommended.[6] The use of screening blood tests is not universally adopted but it is suggested that blood tests should be performed if there is rapidly growing gynaecomastia.[7] A selective policy has also been proposed with blood tests directed at adolescent patients, those with possible endocrine dysfunction or tumours, suspected alcohol excess and patients on long-term medical treatment.[3] If blood tests are performed, they should include renal and liver function tests, follicle simulating hormone, luteinising hormone, thyroid stimulating hormone, lactate dehydrogenase, prolactin, alpha fetoprotein, beta human chorionic gonadotrophin, oestradiol and total testosterone.[7]

Management of Gynaecomastia

Where an underlying cause is identified, this should be corrected where possible. Simple reassurance is often all that is required. Where further treatment is required, the options include medical therapy or surgery. Medical treatments include danazol, tamoxifen, clomifene, which may help to limit the acute proliferative phase, but have limited benefit in chronic established cases. Danazol is the only medication currently licensed for the treatment of gynaecomastia in the UK; however, the evidence for use of these medications is based on small non-randomised trials.[8-10]

The objectives of surgical management are to restore the normal male breast contour with the smallest possible scar. Surgical intervention is usually reserved for Simon's grade IIb and III or gynaecomastia causing significant asymmetry. Surgical options include mastectomy, minimally invasive mastectomy or a combination of the two approaches. There are many techniques for surgical resection and the choice depends on quantity of excess skin. The most common approach is the interareola incision (Webster technique).[11] In severe gynaecomastia, skin resection and nipple transposition techniques may be required, e.g. the Letterman technique,[12] in which the nipple-areola complex is rotated superiorly and medially based on a single dermal pedicle after resection of redundant skin. In massive gynaecomastia, an en bloc resection of excessive skin and breast tissue with free nipple grafting can be performed.

Minimally invasive techniques are increasingly popular. Liposuction, ultrasonic liposuction, arthroscopic shaver and the vacuum-assisted core biopsy device have all been used to perform mastectomy.[13-15] If the gynaecomastia is predominately fatty or pseudogynaecomastia, this technique can be very successful, but it may not be as effective at removing glandular tissue. A combined approach has also been advocated[16] using liposuction initially to remove fatty tissue followed by surgical removal of residual glandular tissue either at a single procedure or a two-staged breast reduction. A technique for liposuction and percutaneous excision using vacuum biopsy for the glandular element has also been described.[17]

MASTALGIA

Breast pain or mastalgia is experienced by most women at some time. It is important to distinguish between true breast pain and referred pain. True breast pain is typically cyclical, worse before menstruation and relieved following menstruation. Referred breast pain is not usually cyclical, often unilateral, associated with activity and may be reproduced by pressure on the chest wall. The cause of true mastalgia is unknown, although research suggests that it may be related to an imbalance in the hormones prolactin and oestrogen.[7] The differential diagnosis for breast pain is broad (Table 5.2). The clinical history may be supplemented by pain charts detailing the severity and timing of the pain. The impact of pain on the patient's life and potential benefit of any treatments should also be established. Physical examination involves exclusion of a discrete breast mass, and of chest wall pain or other non-breast causes of pain including costochondritis medially and lateral chest wall pain. In women over 35 years, a mammogram is usually performed to exclude (occult) malignancy.

TABLE 5.2: Causes of breast pain

Breast related
• Benign breast tumours
• Breast cancer
• Breast cysts
• Breast trauma
• Mastitis
• Sclerosing adenosis
• Thrombophlebitis/Mondor's syndrome
Musculoskeletal
• Cervical and thoracic spondylosis/radiculopathy
• Chest wall trauma and/or rib fracture
• Costochondritis/Tietze's syndrome
• Fibromyalgia
• Herpes zoster
• Shoulder pain
Miscellaneous
• Cholelithiasis/cholecystitis
• Coronary artery disease/angina
• Gastroesophageal reflux
• Medication, e.g. contraceptive pill
• Peptic ulcer disease
• Pericarditis
• Peptic ulcer disease
• Pleurisy
• Pregnancy
• Psychological
• Pulmonary embolus
• Sickle cell anaemia

Management of Mastalgia

Only 2.7% of patients complaining of breast pain are found to have breast cancer,[18] and in many cases, reassurance alone is sufficient with the majority of patients requiring no further treatment. Simple analgesia and a well-fitted bra worn continually may help. For noncyclical breast pain, oral or topical nonsteroidal anti-inflammatory drugs may help. Patients can be advised that cutting out caffeine, a low fat diet and stopping smoking are beneficial, but the scientific evidence for these recommendations is poor. Evening primrose oil (EPO) has commonly been recommended in the past but in 2002, the UK Medicines and Healthcare Products Regulatory Agency withdrew its license due to lack of evidence regarding its effectiveness. Two randomised, crossover trials comparing EPO versus placebo had shown no benefit for EPO,[19,20] and the original evidence advocating the use of EPO was only ever published in abstract form.[21]

More recently, however, a double-blind, randomised, placebo-controlled pilot study carried out at the Mayo clinic showed that EPO alone or in combination with vitamin E may be beneficial in treating breast pain.[22] Starflower oil contains the same active ingredient as EPO (gamma linolenic acid) but in a higher concentration and again can be used for relief of breast pain. Phytoestrogens (e.g. soya milk) and *Agnus castus* (a fruit abstract) may also be of some benefit.[22-24]

Prescribed medication is generally reserved for patients with severe breast pain, and treatment options include danazol and tamoxifen for a limited period, usually 3 months. Trials have suggested that tamoxifen is superior to danazol with fewer adverse effects, although it is not licensed for use in breast pain in the UK. In one study, 53% of patients taking tamoxifen were pain free at 1 year compared to 37% of those on danazol.[25] Higher dose tamoxifen was found to be superior to placebo in a double blind, randomised, controlled trial, with pain relief maintained at 1 year in 72% of patients.[26] A meta-analysis of randomised trials concluded that tamoxifen is associated with fewest side effects and should be the drug of first choice.[27] The adverse effects of these drugs are potentially significant and need to be discussed with the patient. For danazol, these include heavy periods, deepening of voice, acne, hirsutism and weight gain, and for tamoxifen, these include hot flushes, vaginal bleeding, deep vein thrombosis and an increased risk of endometrial cancer. Some of the side effects of tamoxifen may be mitigated by use of a topical preparation (4-hydroxytamoxifen gel),which has shown promise in a phase 2 trial.[28]

> **Key Point**
>
> Tamoxifen is considered the most effective medication for severe breast pain, although this is not a licensed use in the UK. Danazol is a licensed alternative.

NIPPLE DISCHARGE

Nipple discharge accounts for approximately 5% of referrals to a breast clinic. Only 5% of these patients will have malignant disease[18] with the remainder having a physiological cause.

Discharge may be due to duct ectasia, duct papilloma(s), galactorrhoea, ductal carcinoma *in situ* (DCIS), and rarely invasive breast cancer. If there is an associated lump then further management should be directed accordingly. Important features to establish during assessment include frequency of discharge and whether it is blood stained, spontaneous, unilateral or bilateral and from a single or multiple ducts. Features that increase the likelihood that the discharge is due to ductal pathology rather than physiological causes are single duct involvement, or spontaneous, persistent and blood stained, serosanguinous or watery discharge. Galactorrhoea is characterised by bilateral, copious, white multiduct discharge, and can occur a long time after cessation of breastfeeding. Duct ectasia is associated with smoking and is characterised by multiduct, often coloured and bilateral discharge. Clinical assessment for nipple discharge includes careful palpation around the areola to determine if there is a specific location or duct responsible for the discharge.

Investigations

Patients with galactorrhoea should have their prolactin level checked and if raised ($>$ 1,000 mlU/L), this may indicate a pituitary tumour or may be secondary to medication. Breast imaging is usually recommended, with mammography for those over the age of 35 years. Ultrasound may identify a focal dilated duct or intraduct lesion such as a papilloma, or multiple dilated ducts characteristic of duct ectasia. Testing the discharge with a dipstick for haemoglobin determines whether blood is present.

Nipple discharge cytology may be helpful, but has a low sensitivity for detecting malignancy.[29] The presence of profuse or atypical ductal cells may indicate the need for further investigation. Ductal lavage increases cell yield 100 fold, and has been shown to increase sensitivity for malignancy to 64% with a 100% positive predictive value.[30] Ductography can aid detection of ductal lesions and has a sensitivity of around 60% but this is a painful procedure and is not widely or routinely practised.[31]

Ductoscopy is a technique that can be used to investigate nipple discharge. It involves passage of a microendoscope into the respective duct allowing visualisation and the potential for tissue sampling.[32-34] This procedure has been led by developments in technology, with continued miniaturisation of duct endoscopes and continual improvement in the functionality of the optics. Currently its role is predominantly limited to clinical studies, to facilitate targeted surgical excision and potentially to avoid unnecessary surgery.

Management of Nipple Discharge

If examination and imaging do not reveal any abnormality, then simple reassurance or observation may be all that is required. If a patient has spontaneous, single duct, blood-stained discharge that is persistent, then a cause should be found. If a lesion such as a papilloma is identified, it may be suitable for vacuum-assisted core biopsy and percutaneous removal without surgery (see section below). Otherwise the patient should have a needle biopsy followed by image-guided excision assuming the lesion is impalpable. If no cause is found, surgery may be required, since bloody nipple discharge is more frequently associated with ductal carcinoma *in situ* (DCIS) or invasive breast cancer than non-blood-stained nipple discharge.[35] In premenopausal patients, where future breastfeeding may be important, a microdochectomy is often sufficient for diagnosis and treatment, whereas in postmenopausal patients, a major duct excision may be required. Patients with multiduct discharge may be offered major duct excision for symptomatic control.

> **Key Point**
>
> Unilateral, single duct, spontaneous, persistent or blood-stained, serosanguinous or watery nipple discharge are less likely to be physiological and need investigation.

BREAST SEPSIS

Breast sepsis is common and frequently affects women of child-bearing age. Conventionally, breast infection has been categorised into lactational and non-lactational forms. These two groups have differing aetiology, bacteriology, presentation and treatment. Overall 5–33% of women who breastfeed will complain of 'mastitis' at some time, but only a minority will go on to develop a lactational breast abscess (0.4–10%).[36] Lactational abscesses most commonly affect women during the first 6 weeks of breastfeeding or during weaning.[7] Lactational abscesses are usually caused by skin flora such as *Staphylococcus aureus*.[37]

Non-lactational breast abscesses often develop on a background of periductal mastitis (which is predisposed to by smoking) and commonly recurs. Non-lactational abscesses can also be associated with diseases such as diabetes, rheumatoid arthritis, granulomatous lobular mastitis, trauma and steroid treatment. The causal organism again is most commonly *Staphylococcus aureus*, although anaerobic bacteria are frequently involved in addition. The majority of breast abscesses are caused by methicillin-susceptible *Staphylococcus aureus*.[37] The antibiotic of choice should follow local guidelines and should be targeted to any organism identified, but flucloxacillin is often suitable for lactational abscesses. Anaerobic cover may be required for non-lactational abscesses, for example with co-amoxiclav.

Patients with breast sepsis usually present with pain, localised erythema and swelling and may have a fluctuant mass. Pyrexia and leucocytosis are relatively common. Lactational abscesses are often associated with a history of difficulty with breastfeeding, engorgement, poor milk drainage and/or a cracked nipple. If symptoms do not improve with antibiotics, an underlying abscess or drainable collection may be present, which can be diagnosed on ultrasound. Bacteriological cultures should be taken if pus is aspirated. It should be noted that underlying comedo necrosis within DCIS can present as a non-lactational abscess, so patients aged over 35 should have a mammogram when inflammation has settled.[36]

Management of Breast Sepsis

Appropriate management is required to provide symptom control and minimise long-term complications including chronic infection, recurrence and scarring. Numerous reviews and World Health Organization guidelines[38,39] recommend treatment of lactational mastitis with effective milk flow from the engorged segment (by continuation of breastfeeding or breast pump) and antibiotics. Antibiotics used in addition to breast emptying have been shown to clear the patient's symptoms faster than emptying alone (mean 2.1 vs 4.2 days).[39]

Management of Lactational Abscess

Standard management of lactational abscesses remains the use of broad spectrum antibiotics and the drainage of pus. Pus can be aspirated using a wide (14–19) gauge needle, either freehand or under ultrasound guidance; the pus should be sent for microbiological analysis. Vacuum-assisted core biopsy devices have been reported to be of value in some cases. A management algorithm for breast sepsis is shown in Figure 5.2.[40]

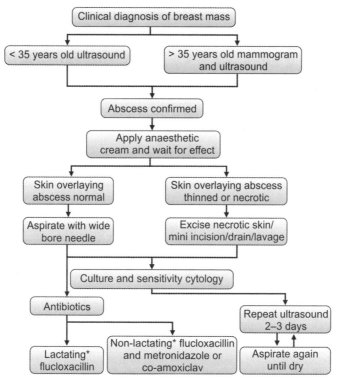

Figure 5.2: Management protocol for breast abscess treatment
Key: * If allergic to penicillin, use alternative antibiotics

The state of the skin overlying the abscess helps determine management. If this skin is thinned or necrotic, a mini-incision (with debridement of any nonviable skin) and drainage should be carried out. This can be performed under local anaesthetic, and rarely requires a general anaesthetic. The cavity should be irrigated with saline until no further pus is present. The patient usually does not require hospital admission unless compromised by systemic sepsis and should be discharged with appropriate antibiotics for review in the breast clinic in the next 2–3 days to ensure adequate resolution of the abscess, or repeat aspiration if indicated.

Most abscesses do not require more than two or three aspirations and patients should be encouraged to continue breastfeeding. If breastfeeding is difficult from the affected breast then the patient should attempt to maintain milk flow with a breast pump until breastfeeding can resume.

If after discussion, the patient wishes to stop breastfeeding then lactation can be suppressed using cabergoline (a dopamine receptor agonist), although side effects can include nausea, vomiting, constipation, dizziness, tiredness and rarely shortness of breath, cough, ankle swelling, mental/mood changes and visual disturbance.

Management of Non-Lactational Abscess

Non-lactational abscesses can be treated in a similar way to lactational abscesses with antibiotics and aspiration or a mini-incision. Smokers who present with a non-lactational abscess should be advised to stop smoking. It is thought that toxins in cigarette smoke damage the walls of ducts, which are then susceptible to infection. There is a reasonably high recurrence rate of non-lactational abscess and up to a third of patients develop a mammary duct fistula following drainage, as aspiration or incision and drainage does not remove the underlying affected ducts. Patients who develop a mammary duct fistula will require excision or laying open of the fistula.[36]

With complex or multiloculated abscesses, ultrasound surface marking of loculi may be helpful in ensuring that all collections are adequately drained. In cases that do not respond in the expected manner, it should be remembered that inflammatory breast cancer is one of the differential diagnoses and tissue biopsy may be required. If standard therapy fails to produce wound healing, vacuum-assisted closure (VAC) therapy can be useful in managing complex chronic wounds.

PERCUTANEOUS MANAGEMENT OF BENIGN BREAST LESIONS

Image-guided core biopsy is considered the standard procedure for obtaining adequate samples of breast tissue for histopathological evaluation in patients with a lesion visible on mammography or ultrasound. Breast core biopsies are typically taken with a 14-gauge device but larger bore vacuum-assisted biopsy/mammotomy devices (VAB/VAM) are increasingly used, enabling the safe and effective acquisition of larger volume specimens. Examination of larger specimens results in reduced potential for underestimation of high-risk lesions and DCIS, increased preoperative diagnosis of breast cancer and decreased rates of diagnostic surgical excision biopsy.[41,42]

In recent years, large bore biopsy has been established as a safe, cost-effective alternative to surgery for the removal of certain benign lesions, particularly fibroadenoma.[41] The usefulness of VAB in the management of benign papillary lesions and radial scars has been demonstrated[42] and there is good evidence that some B3 lesions can be safely managed with percutaneous radiological excision thus avoiding surgical intervention.[43,44]

Large Core Vacuum-Assisted Breast Biopsy and Excision Systems

Two different approaches have been developed for the acquisition of large cores of tissue: multiple contiguous large-bore cores retrieved under suction (VAM) and single very-large-bore core (SLCB). Both types of system are suitable for use in the out patient setting under local anaesthesia.[45]

Vacuum-Assisted Mammotomy Systems

There are four commercially available VAM systems, which are in routine use: the Mammotome, the ATEC, the EnCor and the Vacora. These share basic principles of operation and all allow sampling through 360° through a large bore needle (or probe) but they differ in their design and function. The Vacora takes a single core on each pass and the maximum needle size for this system is 10G. These features limit its usefulness for therapeutic excision biopsy compared with the other systems, which require a single pass to take multiple samples and have maximum needle sizes of 9G (ATEC), 8G (Mammotome) and 7G (EnCor). These devices can be used under stereotactic, ultrasound and magnetic resonance imaging guidance.

Lesions measuring up to 20–30 mm in size are readily removed with VAM, although the EnCor and ATEC systems can retrieve more than 1g of tissue per minute and lesions measuring 50–60 mm in diameter can be excised. Ultrasound is the preferred imaging guidance method whenever possible. Local anaesthetic, usually with adrenaline, is infiltrated into the skin, around the lesion and within the tissues deep to the lesion and a small incision is made in the skin. The probe is introduced, rotating and repositioning it whilst removing multiple samples of tissue until the lesion visible on imaging has been fully removed. Firm pressure is applied to the biopsy site following the procedure to minimise bleeding. The total procedure time may be as little as 15 minutes for small lesions.

Single Large-Core Biopsy System

There is one single large-core radiofrequency (RF) biopsy system in routine use; the intact breast lesion excision system (BLES). This system combines radiofrequency cutting with vacuum to remove a lesion as a complete specimen. Intact BLES may be considered superior to VAM systems as the architecture of both the lesion and surrounding tissue are retained. However, the RF function limits its use in small breasts and for lesions close to the skin or chest wall. The probes (or wands) are available in four sizes to enable retrieval of lesions ranging from 10–20 mm in diameter and the system can be used under stereotactic and ultrasound guidance.

The probe is introduced through a 6–8 mm skin incision following adequate local anaesthesia (as described for VAM biopsy) and advanced to the periphery of the lesion. A cutting RF wire is activated and advanced to cut and ensnare the target within four insulated struts. The single specimen is then removed through the same tract. The effect of RF on the excised sample and surrounding tissues is minimised by the vacuum, which also extracts any blood or haematoma.

Radiological Excision of Fibroadenomas

The evidence supporting radiological excision of fibroadenomas has been assessed and guidance published by the National Institute for Clinical Excellence.[46] Lesions up to 2.5–3 cm in size can be completely removed with minimal or no scarring using a 7- or 8-gauge needle for nodules measuring 1 cm or larger. The rate of successful initial complete removal of a lesion varies widely from 22% to 100% although most studies report rates of 75–100%. Follow-up rates without recurrence are reported at 62–98%.[47]

The procedure is well-tolerated by patients with relatively minor side effects, mainly incomplete excision, haematoma formation and localised infection. A recent study found that in a series of 81 patients undergoing percutaneous vacuum-assisted removal of fibroadenomas with a mean size of 20 mm, pain requiring analgesia persisted for up to 1 week after the procedure in 67%, bruising occurred in 90%, one patient developed a haematoma requiring aspiration and three patients developed minor infections, which resolved with antibiotic therapy.[41]

Radiological Excision of Papillomas

Papillomas are relatively uncommon benign breast neoplasms and are usually detected as an asymptomatic mass or calcification, or may present with nipple discharge, bleeding from the nipple or a palpable mass. The majority of solitary papillomas are benign, but there is a risk of associated atypia or malignancy (with some papers quoting the level of risk at over 30%). For this reason, management has conventionally involved surgical excision to enable a confident diagnosis of benign papilloma to exclude associated malignancy in the adjacent parenchyma and to prevent subsequent malignant change within the lesion. However, vacuum-assisted excision under ultrasound guidance is now considered an appropriate alternative approach with subsequent surgical excision only in cases where atypia or malignancy are found (Fig. 5.3).[43,48] The risk of recurrence of solitary papillomas after surgical or vacuum-assisted excision has not been well documented although recurrence was reported in 3 of 26 and 2 of 13 cases of benign papilloma following vacuum-assisted removal,[43,49] and use of a 7G or 8G probe may therefore be recommended for all but the smallest lesions.

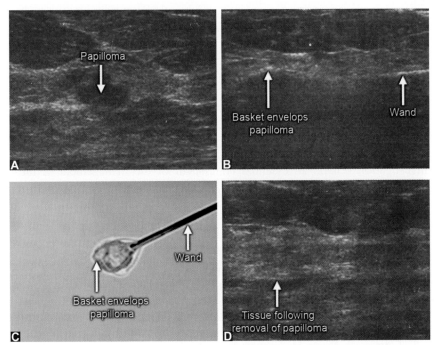

Figures 5.3A to D: Percutaneous excision of a papilloma under ultrasound guidance Identification of the papilloma by ultrasound (A). The percutaneous device is inserted under ultrasound guidance and the basket deployed to envelop the papilloma (B, and schematically C). Images A, B and D are kindly provided by Drs Ali Sever and Karina Cox, Maidstone and Tunbridge Wells NHS Trust. Image C is reproduced from *Intact Sales Aid 2005* with kind permission

Radiological Excision of Radial Scars

Vacuum-assisted excision may also have a role in the management of radial scars in which no atypia has been demonstrated on multiple VAB cores. Carcinoma in radial scars under 6–7 mm in size is very uncommon, but the risk increases with increasing size.[50] Foci of atypical and malignant changes are also often small and may comprise as little as 5% of the lesion,[51] hence the risk of sampling error. It has therefore been proposed that optimal management for radial scars exceeding 10 mm in size still requires diagnostic surgical excision biopsy.[44]

> **Key Point**
>
> Vacuum-assisted biopsy/mammotomy devices can be safely used as an alternative to surgical excision of solitary breast papillomas, small fibroadenomas and radial scars under 10 mm.

CONCLUSION

The management of benign breast conditions continues to evolve and constitutes an important component of the symptomatic breast clinic. Whilst technology has enabled less invasive approaches to many of the conditions, such as liposuction for gynaecomastia, ultrasound-guided aspiration for breast sepsis and radiological excision of benign breast lesions, careful clinical assessment and investigation remain an essential component of the management of these conditions.

> **Key Points**
>
> 1. Tamoxifen is considered the most effective medication for severe breast pain, although this is not a licensed use in the UK. Danazol is a licensed alternative.
> 2. Unilateral, single duct, spontaneous, persistent or blood-stained, serosanguinous or watery nipple discharge are less likely to be physiological and need investigation.
> 3. Vacuum-assisted biopsy/mammotomy devices can be safely used as an alternative to surgical excision of solitary breast papillomas, small fibroadenomas and radial scars under 10 mm.

REFERENCES

1. Nydick M, Bustos J, Dale JH, et al. Gynaecomastia in adolescent boys. JAMA. 1961;178:(5):449-54.
2. Glass AR. Gynaecomastia. Endocrinol Metab Clin North Am. 1994;23(4):825-37.
3. Simon BE, Hoffman S, Kahn S. Classification and surgical correction of gynaecomastia. Plast Reconstr Surg. 1973;51:48-52.
4. Rahmani S, Turton P, Shaaban A, et al. Overview of gynaecomastia in the modern era and the Leeds gynaecomastia investigation algorithm. Breast J. 2011;17(3):246-55.
5. Carrasco R, Benito M, Gomariz E, et al. Mammography and ultrasound in the evaluation of male breast disease. Eur Radiol. 2010;20:2797-805.
6. Janes SE, Lengyel JA, Singh S, et al. Needle core biopsy for the assessment of unilateral breast masses in men. Breast. 2006;15:273-5.
7. Thrush S, Dixon M. Companion series: Breast Disease. 2009, Chapter 17, 259-79.
8. Jones DJ, Holt SD, Surtees P, et al. A comparison of danazol and placebo in the treatment of adult idiopathic gynaecomastia: results of a prospective study in 55 patients. Ann R Coll Surg Engl. 1990;72:296-8.
9. Khan HN, Blamey RW. Endocrine treatment of physiological gynaecomastia. Br Med J. 2003;327:301-2.
10. Plourde P, Kulin H, Santner SJ. Clomiphene in the treatment of adolescent gynaecomastia. Clinical and endocrine studies. Am J Dis Child. 1983;137:1080-2.
11. Webster DJ. The male breast. Br J Clin Pract Suppl. 1989;68:137-42.
12. Letterman G, Schurter M. A comparison of modern methods of reduction mammaplasty. South Med J. 1976;69:1367-71.
13. Jarrar G, Peel A, Fahmy H, et al. Single incision endoscopic surgery for gynaecomastia. J Plast Reconstr Aesthet Surg. 2011;64:e231-6.
14. Petty PM, Solomon M, Buchel EW, et al. Gynaecomastia: evolving paradigm of management and comparison of techniques. Plast Reconstr Surg. 2011;125:1301-8.
15. He Q, Zheng L, Zhuang D, et al. Surgical treatment of gynaecomastia by vacuum-assisted biopsy device. J Laparoendosc Adv Surg Tech A. 2011;21(5):431-4.

16. Esme DL, Beekman WH, Hage JJ, et al. Combined use of ultrasonic-assisted liposuction and semicircular periareolar incision for the treatment of gynaecomastia. Ann Plast Surg. 2007;59(6):629-34.

17. Qutob O, Elahi B, Garimella V, et al. Minimally invasive excision of gynaecomastia—a novel and effective surgical technique. Ann R Coll Surg Eng. 2010;92(3):198-200.

18. Mansel RE. ABC of breast diseases. Breast pain. Br Med J. 1994;309:866-8.

19. Khoo SK, Munro C, Battistutta D. Evening primrose oil and treatment of premenstrual syndrome. Med J Aust. 1990;153:189-92.

20. Blommers J, de Lange-De Klerk E, Kuik D, et al. Evening primrose oil and fish oil for severe chronic mastalgia: a randomized, double blind controlled trial. Am J Obstet Gynaecol. 2002;187:1389-94.

21. Pashby N, Mansel R, Hughes L, et al. A clinical trial of evening primrose oil in mastalgia. Br J Surg. 1981;68:801-24.

22. Pruthi S, Wahner-Roedler D, Torkelson CJ, et al. Vitamin E and evening primrose oil for management of cyclical mastalgia: a randomized pilot study. Altern Med Rev. 2011;15(1):59-66.

23. McFayden I, Chetty U, Setchell K, et al. A randomised double blind crossover trial of soya protein for the treatment of cyclical breast pain. Breast. 2000;9:271-6.

24. Halaska M, Raus K, Beles P, et al. Treatment of cyclical mastodynia using an extract of *Vitex agnus-castus*: results of a double-blind comparison with a placebo. Ceska Gynekol. 1998;63:388-92.

25. Kontostolis E, Stefanidis K, Navrozoglou I, et al. Comparison of tamoxifen with danazol for treatment of cyclical mastalgia. Gynecol Endocrinol. 1997;11:393-7.

26. Fentiman IS, Caleffi M, Brame K, et al. Double-blind controlled trial of tamoxifen therapy for mastalgia. Lancet. 1986;1:287-8.

27. Srivastava A, Mansel RE, Arvind N, et al. Evidence-based management of mastalgia: a meta-analysis of randomised trials. Breast. 2007;16:503-12.

28. Mansel R, Goyal A, Nestour EL, et al. A phase II trial of Afimoxifene (4-hydroxytamoxifen gel) for cyclical mastalgia in premenopausal women. Breast Cancer Res Treat. 2007;106:389-97.

29. Simmons R, Adamovich T, Brennan M, et al. Nonsurgical evaluation of pathologic nipple discharge. Ann Surg Oncol. 2003;10:113-16.

30. Shen K, Wu J, Lu J, et al. Fiberoptic ductoscopy for breast cancer patients with nipple discharge. Surg Endosc. 2001;15:1340-5.

31. King BL, Love SM, Rochman S, et al. The Fourth International Symposium on the Intraductal Approach to Breast Cancer, Santa Barbara, California, 10-13 March 2005. Breast Cancer Res. 2005;7(5):198-204.

32. Tang SS, Twelves DJ, Isacke CM, et al. Mammary ductoscopy in the current management of breast disease. Surg Endosc. 2011;25(6):1712-22.

33. Kamali S, Bender O, Aydin MT, et al. Ductoscopy in the evaluation and management of nipple discharge. Ann Surg Oncol. 2010;17(3):778-83.

34. Vaughan A, Crowe J, Brainard J, et al. Mammary ductoscopy and ductal washings for the evaluation of patients with pathologic nipple discharge. Breast J. 2009;15(3):254-60.

35. Chen L, Zhou WB, Zhao Y, et al. Bloody nipple discharge is a predictor of breast cancer risk: a meta-analysis. Breast Cancer Res Treat. 2012;132:9-14.

36. Dixon JM, Khan LR. Treatment of breast infection. BMJ. 2011;342:342-489.

37. Dabbas N, Chand M, Pallett A, et al. Have the organisms that cause breast abscess changed with time? Implications for appropriate antibiotic usage in primary and secondary care. Breast J. 2010;16(4):412-5.

38. World Health Organization. (2000). Mastitis: causes and management. [online] Available from http://www.who.int/maternal_child_adolescent/documents/fch_cah_00_13/en/ [Accessed August, 2012].

39. Jahanfar S, Ng CJ, Teng CL. Antibiotics for mastitis in breastfeeding women. Cochrane Database Syst Rev. 2009;CD005458.

40. Agrawal A, Kissen M. Breast abscess. Br J Hosp Med (Lond). 2007;68(11):M198-9.

41. Thurley P, Evans A, Hamilton L, et al. Patient satisfaction and efficacy of vacuum-assisted excision biopsy of fibroadenomas. Clin Radiol. 2009;64,381-5.

42. Tennant SL, Evans A, Hamilton LJ, et al. Vacuum-assisted excision of breast lesions of uncertain malignant potential (B3) - an alternative to surgery in selected cases. Breast. 2008;17:546-9.

43. Maxwell AJ. Ultrasound-guided vacuum-assisted excision of breast papillomas: review of 6-years experience. Clin Radiol. 2009;64:801-6.

44. Rajan S, Shaaban AM, Dall BJ, et al. New patient pathway using vacuum-assisted biopsy reduces diagnostic surgery for B3 lesions. Clin Radiol. 2012;67:244-9.

45. Brun del Re, Renzo (Ed.) Minimally Invasive Breast Biopsies. New York: Springer-Verlag; 2009. pp. 23-40.

46. National Institute for Health and Clinical Excellence. (2006). Interventional Procedure Guidance 156. Image-guided vacuum-assisted excision biopsy of benign breast lesions. [online]. Available from http://www.nice.org.uk/nicemedia/live/11210/31513/31513.pdf. [Accessed August 2012].

47. Park HL, Kim LS. The current role of vacuum-assisted breast biopsy system in breast disease. J Breast Cancer. 2011;14(1):1-7.

48. Kim MJ, Kim SI, Youk JH, et al. The diagnosis of non-malignant papillary lesions of the breast: comparison of ultrasound-guided automated gun biopsy and vacuum-assisted removal. Clin Radiol. 2011;66:530-5.

49. Bonaventure T, Cormier B, Lebas P, et al. Benign papilloma: is US-guided vacuum-assisted breast biopsy an alternative to surgery? J Radiol. 2007;88:1165-8.

50. Sloane JP, Mayers MM. Carcinoma and atypical hyperplasia in radial scars and complex sclerosing lesions: importance of lesion size and patient age. Histopathology. 1993;23:225-31.

51. Farshid G, Rush G. Assessment of 142 stellate lesions with imaging features suggestive of radial scar discovered during population-based screening for breast cancer. Am J Surg Pathol. 2004;28:1626-31.

6

Management of Facial Paralysis

D Bray

INTRODUCTION

Significant functional, aesthetic and psychosocial sequelae accompany facial paralysis. Dysfunctional lacrimation, palpebral fissure widening, loss of blink reflex and orbicularis function can lead to exposure keratopathy and corneal ulceration. Lagophthalmos is potentiated by paralytic eyelid, ectropion, and upper and lower lid retraction. The absent lower lid and nasal twist further exaggerates epiphora.[1]

The loss of oral competence leads to drooling and articulation difficulty. Nasal alar collapse, nasolabial flattening and nasal valve dysfunction add further to the social stigma associated with the induced nasal speech. The psychological impact of facial disfigurement and unwelcome attention is profound resulting in depression, agoraphobia and social isolation.[2]

Rehabilitation of the paralysed face presents a complex and challenging management problem. Potential for nerve regeneration varies widely and as yet, accurate prognostic indicators of spontaneous recovery do not exist. This directly influences the decision regarding reanimation as certain techniques interfere with or even preclude the normal recovery process. Facial function and appearance can be improved with physical therapy, botulinum toxin injection and surgery. Surgical options include primary neurorrhaphy, interpositional nerve grafts, nerve substitution techniques, static resuspension and/or dynamic reanimation. The cause of paralysis and degree of functional impairment, as well as the patient's age and medical history must be considered before any intervention. Adequate observation time from onset of paralysis, and appropriate patient and procedure selection is paramount to achieve the best surgical outcome.

During the past century, approaches to reanimation of the paralysed face have seen the development and refinement of surgical techniques to restore dynamic function via regional muscle transposition,[3] free muscle transfer[4,5] and more recently, muscle lengthening procedures.[6,7]

Long-term goals of facial reanimation are to achieve normal appearance at rest, symmetrical movement and restoration of voluntary muscle control.[8]

NEURAL TECHNIQUES

Primary Neurorrhaphy

Primary end-to-end anastomosis of the facial nerve at the time of injury is the most effective method of rehabilitating the paralysed face. This is relevant in iatrogenic injury during oncological resection or prompt surgical intervention after temporal bone fracture or sharp trauma to the branchiomotor division. The repair is best achieved at, or within 30 days of, the primary ablative operation. The limiting factors for primary neurorrhaphy are access to the intracranial facial nerve and sufficient neuronal length.

The present neurorrhaphy technique uses a microscope, specialised microinstrumentation and the use of 8-0/10-0 monofilament suture. When the ends of the injured facial nerve have been identified, they are trimmed, and the epineurium is peeled back to expose the endoneurium. One percent methylene blue is applied to the exposed nerve ends with a cotton-tipped applicator. The epineural sheath stains dark blue whilst the endoneurial surface stains a lighter blue facilitating accurate approximation.[9] One or two perineural sutures between the proximal and distal nerve trunks usually suffice. A tension-free anastomosis is essential to prevent scar formation and subsequent disruption of axonal regeneration.[10] If tension-free neurorrhaphy cannot be achieved, mobilisation of the neural segments or interpositional grafts may be necessary.

Interpositional Grafts

When a tension-free anastomosis cannot be achieved with primary neurorrhaphy, or facial nerve length has been sacrificed to obtain tumour clearance in oncologic resection, several donor nerves are available for interpositional grafting. The greater auricular and sural nerves, however, are most suitable for facial nerve repair in terms of their availability, axonal content and length.[28] They are also readily accessible, and the area of sensory deficit created by their harvest is acceptable to the patient. The length of the graft should be at least 1–2 mm longer than the gap it is to bridge to ensure a tension-free anastomosis. In the adult, upto 10 cm of the greater auricular nerve can be harvested. It is found by bisecting at right angles, a line drawn between the mastoid tip and angle of the mandible, and is easily accessible at neck dissection. The sural nerve has three advantages over the greater auricular nerve. First, a greater length can be obtained (upto 40 cm), second, it has a greater number of neural fascicles, and third, it will not be involved in the primary oncological resection. The sural nerve lies between the lateral malleolus and the Achilles tendon, 1 cm lateral and deep to the saphenous vein. Nerve harvest using multiple transverse incisions decreases postoperative pain on ambulation and avoids the unsightly scar that follows long vertical incision. The technique for neuronal anastomosis is as described above, and the expected rate of axonal regeneration is 1 mm/ day. Patients can expect to have adequate facial tone after 6 months and restoration of motion 1–3 months thereafter.[10]

Cranial Nerve Crossover

Using other cranial nerves for facial reanimation should be considered when the proximal central stump is unavailable, primary nerve grafts are not possible, and surgery can be performed within 2 years of injury. This is most commonly seen following nerve sacrifice, cerebellopontine angle tumour surgery, radical oncologic resection of the temporal bone, parotid and skull base, and severe temporal bone brainstem trauma. Various options include classic hypoglossal facial anastomosis, hypoglossal facial jump grafting and facial nerve cross facial anastomosis. The main disadvantage of donor nerve techniques is the inevitable sacrifice in donor cranial nerve function. Complete transection of the hypoglossal nerve leads to ipsilateral paralysis and hemitongue atrophy, causing difficulty with mastication, speech and swallowing. Functional disability is variable. Pensak et al noted that 74% of patients reported some difficulty with eating, whilst only 21% found it debilitating. Rarely was swallowing significantly disturbed, and although articulation was affected in all patients initially, rarely was this disabling and improvement was significant over time. Interestingly, whilst mid and lower facial reanimation was satisfactory to the patient, 75% reported incomplete eye closure, and of these, 21% developed ophthalmic sequelae.[11] It is therefore advisable to combine this technique with ophthalmic reanimation and/or protection as discussed later. May and Drucker described the hypoglossal-facial interposition jump graft[12] for use in patients with bilateral facial paralysis, other cranial nerve deficits (a combined X and XII deficit risks aspiration on swallowing), in those with neurofibromatosis Type 2, and in those who refuse to accept the sequelae of unilateral hypoglossal palsy. This procedure involves partially incising rather than transecting the hypoglossal nerve. Sufficient numbers of hypoglossal axons remain to spare tongue function whilst axonal regeneration can occur across an interposition end-to-side 'jump' graft anastomosed to the distal ipsilateral facial stump to reanimate the paralysed face (an indirect hypoglossal-facial anastomosis). Manni et al[13] followed up 39 patients who underwent indirect hypoglossal-facial anastomosis. All patients had normal tongue function, and most achieved House Brackman grade III (44.6%), II (20.9%) or IV (24.1%) (House Brackman grading is the globally accepted facial palsy grading scale).

Whilst this technique preserves ipsilateral tongue function with two anastomoses, the return of facial nerve motor function is inevitably slower and weaker when compared with direct hypoglossal-facial anastomosis. To address this, Atlas and Lowinger[14] modified the technique in three patients by connecting the distal facial nerve directly to a partially incised hypoglossal nerve. Sufficient length was achieved by removing the mastoid tip. The facial nerve was mobilised in the temporal bone, sectioned at the second genu, and following transposition from the mastoid segment, an end-to-side hypoglossal anastomosis was performed. Although only small numbers have been described, all patients achieved a highly satisfactory cosmetic and functional outcome.

Cross-face grafting (facial-facial anastomosis) was originally described by Scaramella.[15] A crossed facial nerve graft is used to extend the buccal nerve branch of the animated facial nerve across the upper lip by the alar base (Fisch's modification)[16] to the contralateral distal facial nerve. The obvious disadvantage of this procedure is the sacrifice of normal facial function for the potential benefit to the paralysed side. The more distal the donor branched used, the less axonal flow; the more proximal, the greater the donor deficit. May and Schaitkin, therefore, suggest that cross-face grafting should not be used as a primary procedure, but should be used to power a free muscle graft or to augment other procedures that are performed to restore facial function.[17]

REGIONAL MUSCLE TRANSPOSITION

There are three regional muscles available for reanimation. The temporalis muscle, used for perioral reanimation (upper/lower lip, melolabial fold and alar base) is the most popular due to its length, location, contractility and vector of pull to restore the position of the corner of the mouth to create a lateral smile. The masseter muscle is less frequently used because it provides an unphysiological horizontal action on the lip commissure, an unaesthetic depression over the mandibular angle and longer-term mastication difficulty. It may be useful as an adjunct to temporalis muscle transposition or following radical parotid surgery. The digastric muscle is transposed to partially restore function following the loss of depressor anguli oris innervated by the marginal mandibular branch of the facial nerve.

The temporalis muscle is animated by the trigeminal nerve, and is unresponsive to emotion without extensive retraining. The voluntary, balanced lateral smile therefore, may be achieved only in the well-motivated patient willing to work, often for a long period, with a specialist physiotherapist. A major advantage of temporalis muscle transposition is the possibility to reanimate partial facial function, or in those patients where some facial nerve recovery is expected. The facial nerve lies deep to the superficial musculoaponeurotic system (SMAS), so the muscle can be transposed through a tunnel superficial to the SMAS without disturbing the facial nerve fibres. The procedure therefore, can be performed at the same time as a nerve repair or XII-VII crossover to give an immediate improvement, that in no way compromises the outcome of the nerve repair. The main disadvantages of temporalis transposition are lack of spontaneous movement, chronic temporomandibular joint dysfunction and tissue bulk over the zygomatic arch.[18]

An exciting recent development, the lengthening temporalis myoplasty, described by Labbé[6] addresses several disadvantages. In his article, Labbé improves on McLaughlin's original technique[19] by transferring the temporalis tendon, still attached to the coronoid process, directly to the lips. He performs a true myoplasty without the need for an intermediate fascia lata graft. The fixed temporal point is preserved on the anterior temporal crest, and the lengthened temporalis passes deep to the zygomatic arch, thereby eradicating the unaesthetic zygomatic bulge/temporal hollow previously seen. Stretching the muscle results in an immediate overcorrection, which is necessary to allow for normal muscle attenuation. Intraoral contralateral myectomies may afford better symmetry;[20] however, this can be achieved with Botox® injection. Byrne et al recently reviewed their experience with this technique and concluded that patient satisfaction was high; the procedure was relatively easy to perform, minimally invasive and eliminated the facial asymmetry typical of temporalis transfer.[7]

FREE MUSCLE TRANSFER

The aim of free muscle transfer for facial reanimation is to achieve a natural and subconscious smile. It is indicated when native facial muscles are absent, denervated for greater than 2-years duration, or when regional muscles have been damaged by oncologic resection or tumour. Harii et al in 1973 successfully transferred the gracilis to the face with both neural and vascular anastomoses, and demonstrated subsequent functional reinnervation.[4] Since then, a variety of muscles have been used for free tissue transfer, but the most popular in descending order of frequency are the gracilis, pectoralis minor and latissimus dorsi. The criteria for selection of a muscle include fibre length commensurate with zygomaticus major, 6–8 cm in length, suitable vascular architecture, location and structure of suitable tendinous anchor points and a donor nerve of sufficient length to reach the ipsilateral hypoglossal nerve or previous cross-face nerve transfer. The sacrifice of the donor muscle must not lead to significant donor site morbidity. In a study of various muscles available, Terzis found that the pectoralis minor was most suitable for these criteria. The pectoralis minor also has a high density of motor nerve axons available for reanimation—a 'smart muscle'.[21] This preference for pectoralis minor is supported by Harrison,[5] but in a recent cadaveric study, Bove et al assessed suitability of flaps in terms of microsurgical (vascular pedicle size and diameter), anatomical (thickness, fibre direction) and functional characteristics (power, extensibility), and concluded that the most suitable to flap was the latissimus dorsi, followed by gracilis then pectoralis minor.[22] Whichever donor muscle is used, reinnervation restores facial tone at 4–5 months and movement can be expected after 7–8 months.[23]

Selection of the donor nerve to innervate the free graft depends on the aetiology of facial paralysis, availability of functioning ipsilateral facial nerve, previous facial surgery and patient preference. Options include using the original proximal facial nerve after oncologic resection (often from within the fallopian canal), the contralateral facial nerve via a cross-face sural nerve graft in a two-stage procedure, and the ipsilateral hypoglossal nerve. The latter may achieve some degree of voluntary smile by pressing the tongue on to the hard palate, but will not achieve the involuntary mimetic innervation of the free graft seen when the facial nerve is used.

OPHTHALMIC PROTECTION AND REHABILITATION

Orbital protection and subsequent rehabilitation are mandatory in facial palsy. A comprehensive review of oculoplastic techniques, such as that published recently by Rahman and Sadiq,[24] falls outside the scope of this chapter, but the common interventions have been discussed.

Conservative Orbital Protection

Protection of the exposed cornea, and close monitoring and treatment of corneal complications is the primary concern. The lower-third of the cornea is most often affected dependent on the degree of lagophthalmos. If recovery of facial function is expected, conservative measures are best adopted with meticulous monitoring.

Lubrication with methylcellulose preparations is necessary, drops during the daytime and more viscous ointment at night, with taping or patching to prevent nocturnal inadvertent trauma. Moisture chambers have been used with good effect. Patients lubricate the eye before applying a Cartella shield with an overlying cellophane dressing. This acts as orbital 'greenhouse' retaining moisture within the pocket. In patients with reduced tear production or in whom lubrication and patching fails to address corneal exposure, punctal occlusion with punctal plugs may be successful.

Botulinum Toxin

Botox® (Allergan, Berks) provides good corneal protection by inducing a protective ptosis by temporarily paralysing levator palpebrae superioris. In one series of 21 patients, the induced ptosis was sustained for a mean of 46 days following onset after 4 days.[25] Another study reported a 45% rate of temporary diplopia, but advocated Botox® use as eyelid scarring is avoided, topical therapy may be continued and corneal examination was possible.[26]

Corneal Protective Surgery

These days, surgical measures to ensure corneal protection in the acute phase are less frequent employed. Tarsorrhaphy has been superceded by other rehabilitative procedures such as suborbicularis oculi fat lifts (SOOF lifts), lid loading and canthoplasty. Tarsorrhaphy has been criticized for its lack of peripheral vision, poor cosmesis and ineffectiveness. It is best reserved for those patients in whom medical therapy is difficult, lacrimal gland function is lost, or in combined V/VII nerve paresis where corneal sensation is impaired. Upper lid loading was first introduced in the 1950s,[27] and has stood the test of time. Weighting of the upper lid results in an increased gravitational pull of on the lid, and aided by levator palpebrae relaxation, the paralysed eyelid may close passively, greatly reducing lagophthalmos. Gold, first suggested in 1966, is now standard, but Berghaus et al[28] suggest that linked platinum may have superior characteristics. A smaller volume is required due to the greater density of platinum (21.5 g/cm^3) when compared with gold (19.4 g/cm^3); the flexible chain linkage allows for better contour to the tarsal plate, and on histological examination of the peri-implant capsule, less inflammation was observed.

In the longer term, after an initial waiting period for return of normal facial function, oculoplastic surgery in the form of canthoplasty, lid shortening procedures and lower lid spacers (with conchal[29] or auricular cartilage[30] grafts) should coincide with correction of the ptotic mid-facial region. Lisman demonstrated superior lower lid reanimation once the paralytic mid-facial region had been elevated.[31] The extent of gravitational ectropion is dependent on the laxity allowed by the tarsal plate and the medial and lateral canthal tendons. The procedure of choice, therefore, requires an individualised approach to obtain the best functional and cosmetic result.

ADJUNCTIVE TECHNIQUES

Botulinum toxin is the simplest method of providing symmetry by paralysing the contralateral hyperfunctioning muscles. This is most marked in isolated marginal mandibular paralysis with chemical denervation of the contralateral depressor labii inferioris (DLI). Hussain et al[32] reported a 93% (39/42) success rate with contralateral DLI resection resulting in improved aesthetic lower lip symmetry at rest and on animation. The effect was mimicked preoperatively with selective DLI Botox® injection. Care needs to be taken to avoid oral incompetence to fluids or food, which has been reported to occur as frequently as 50% and 17%, respectively in a recent study.[33]

Facial slings can improve facial symmetry and function in those who are medically unfit, or wish to undergo reanimation surgery. Whilst donor site morbidity and foreign body reactions with autologous fascia lata have been reduced with the advent of synthetic expanded polytetrafluoroethylene (Gore-Tex, WL Gore, Flagstaff AZ), and allografts such as human acellular dermis (Alloderm, Lifecell Corp. Branchberg NJ), late complications leading to revision surgery are not uncommon.[34] All are used successfully to lift the mid-and lower-atonic facial musculature. A multivectored suture sling technique has recently been described.[35] Perioral and perialar 3/0 permanent sutures are passed deep to midfacial soft tissues with a Keith needle and anchored through lateral orbital wall drill holes. The procedure has distinct advantages over standard static sling techniques; however, the medium- and long-term resilience of this technique has not been demonstrated. The multivector system accounts for the different vectors of pull of normal facial musculature, the technique requires small incisions and can therefore be performed under local anaesthesia enabling patient assistance by contralateral facial movement, and small changes and adjustments can be made in the outpatient clinic.

Facial rejuvenation surgery, including SMAS and MACS (Minimal Access Cranial Suspension) rhytidectomy, blepharoplasty and endoscopic browlift techniques, can improve the functional and cosmetic deficit in facial paralysis patients. The lateral pull of rhytidectomy has been shown to improve nasal valve function on acoustic rhinometry.[36]

THE FUTURE

It is an exciting time in the realm of facial paralysis management. Technological advances in digital photography and laser facial mapping are enabling development of tools to objectively evaluate facial movement and function.[37] Once this tool is available and standardised, a web-based data archive will provide quantitative validated outcome measures for current treatment strategies and enable a global consensus.[38] Research progresses in the field of nerve regeneration. Future work is likely to focus on improving axonal growth along nerve grafts and improving target accuracy.[39] High efficiency transmission of axons through nerve grafting material is likely to involve 'smart' biomaterials in which both polymeric substances and biologically relevant agents are combined to create living bioartificial nerve conduits.[40]

CONCLUSION

Whilst there have been significant advances in, and refinement of surgical technique for rehabilitation of the paralysed face in recent years, we have yet to achieve a consensus for surgical management. The cause of this is multifactorial and includes patient specific factors and physician preference. What is agreed upon, however, is that the facial paralysis patient requires a detailed physical, functional and psychological evaluation. The treatment choices are based on the cause and duration of paralysis, and the patient's condition and expectations of outcome. The choice of therapy can be overwhelming to the patient, but it is essential that they are engaged in the decision making process. Any intervention undertaken, be it surgery or physiotherapy, will require absolute dedication, compliance and endurance to achieve the best outcome.

REFERENCES

1. Arrigg P, Miller D. A new lid sign in seventh nerve palsy. Ann Ophthalmol. 1985;17:43-5.
2. Bradbury ET, Simons W, Sanders R. Psychological and social factors in reconstructive surgery for hemi-facial palsy. J Plast Reconstr Aesthet Surg. 2006;59(3):272-8.
3. Erlacher P. Direct and muscular neurotization of paralysed muscles. Am J Ortho Surg. 1915;13:22-32.
4. Harii K, Ohmori K, Torii S. Free gracilis muscle transplantation, with microneurovascular anastomoses for the treatment of facial paralysis. A preliminary report. Plast Reconstr Surg. 1976;57:133-43.
5. Harrison DH. The pectoralis minor vascularised muscle graft for the treatment of unilateral facial palsy. Plast Reconstr Surg. 1985;75:206-16.
6. Labbe D, Huault M. Lengthening temporalis myoplasty and lip reanimation. Plast Reconstr Surg. 2000;105(4):1289-97.
7. Byrne PJ, Kim M, Boahene K, et al. Temporalis tendon transfer as part of a comprehensive approach to facial reanimation. Arch Facial Plast Surg. 2007;9(4):234-41.
8. Cheney ML, Mckenna MJ, Nath R, et al. Facial nerve reconstruction and facial reanimation following oncologic surgery. Head Neck. 1999;21(3):276-84.
9. May M, Schaitkin BM (Eds). The Facial Nerve. May's second edition. New York: Thieme. p. 572.
10. Schindo M. Management of facial nerve paralysis. Otolaryngol Clin North Am. 1999;32:945-64.
11. Pensak ML, Jackson GG, Glasscock ME, et al. Facial reanimation with the VII-XII anastomosis: analysis of the functional and physiological results. Otolaryogol Head Neck Surg. 1986;94:305-10.
12. May M, Drucker C. Temporalis muscle for facial reanimation. A 13-year experience with 224 procedures. Arch Otolaryngol Head Neck Surg. 1993;119:378-82.
13. Manni JJ, Beurskens CH, van de Velde C, et al. Reanimation of the paralysed face by indirect hypoglossal-facial nerve anastomosis. Am J Surg. 2001;182:268-273.
14. Atlas MD, Lowinger DS. A new technique for hypoglossal-facial nerve repair. Laryngoscope. 1997;107:984-991.
15. Scaramella LF. Preliminary report on facial nerve anastomosis. Second International Symposium on Facial Nerve Surgery, Osaka, Japan, 1970.
16. Fisch U. Facial nerve grafting. Otolaryngol Clin North Am. 1974;7:517-29.
17. May M, Schaitkin BM (Eds). The Facial Nerve. May's second edition. New York: Thieme. p. 627.
18. Conley J, Baker DC, Selfe RW. Paralysis of the mandibular branch of the facial nerve. Plast Reconstr Surg. 1982;70:569-77.
19. McLaughlin CR. Surgical support in permanent facial paralysis. Plast Reconstr Surg. 1953;11:302-14.
20. Niklison J. Facial paralysis: moderation of non-paralysed muscles. Br J Plast Surg. 1965;18:397-405.
21. Terzis JK. Pectoralis minor: a unique muscle for correction of facial paralysis. Plast Reconstr Surg. 1989;83:767-76.
22. Bove A, Chiarini S, D'Andrea V, et al. Facial nerve palsy: which flap? Microsurgical, anatomical, and functional considerations. Microsurgery 1998;18:286-89.
23. Shindo M. Facial reanimation with microneurovasular free flaps. Facial Plast Surg. 2000;16:357-9.

24. Rahman I, Sadiq SA. Ophthalmic management of facial palsy: a review. Surv Ophthalmol. 2007;52(2):121-44.
25. Ellis MF, Daniell M. An evaluation of the safety and efficacy of botulinum toxin type A (Botox) when used to produce a protective ptosis. Clin Experiment Ophthalmol. 2001;29:394-9.
26. Sadiq SA, Downes RN: A clinical algorithm for the management is facial nerve palsy from an oculoplastic perspective. Eye. 1998;12(2):219-23.
27. Sheehan, JE. Progress in correction of facial plasy with tantalum wire and mesh. Surgery. 1950;27:122-5.
28. Berghaus A, Neumann K, Schrom T. The platinum chain: a new upper-lid implant for facial palsy. Arch Facial Plast Surg. 2003;5:166-70.
29. Jackson IT, Dubin B, Harris J. Use of contoured and stabilized conchal cartilage grafts for lower eyelid support: a preliminary report. Plast Reconstr Surg. 1989;83:636-40.
30. May M, Hoffmann DF, Buerger GF, et al. Management of the paralyzed lower eyelid by implanting auricular cartilage. Arch Otolaryngol Head Neck Surg. 1990;116:786-8.
31. Lisman RD, Smith B, Baker D, et al. Efficacy of surgical treatment for paralytic ectropion. Ophthalmology. 1987;94:671-81.
32. Hussain G, Manktelow RT, Tomat LR. Depressor labii inferioris resection: an effective treatment for marginal mandibular nerve paralysis. Br J Plast Surg. 2004;57:502-10.
33. de Maio M, Bento RF. Botulinum toxin in facial palsy: an effective treatment for contralateral hyperkinesis. Plast Reconstr Surg. 2007;120(4):917-27.
34. Constantinides M, Galli SK, Miller PJ. Complications of static facial suspensions with expanded polytetrafluoroethylene (ePTFE). Laryngoscope. 2001;111(12):2114-21.
35. Alex JC, Nguyen DB. Multivectored suture suspension: a minimally invasive technique for reanimation of the paralyzed face. Arch Facial Plast Surg. 2004;6:197-201.
36. Capone RB, Sykes JM. The effect of rhytidectomy on the nasal valve. Arch Facial Plast Surg. 2005;7:45-50.
37. Frey M, Giovanoli P, Gerber H, et al. Three-dimensional video analysis of facial movements: a new method to assess the quantity and quality of the smile. Plast Reconstr Surg. 1999;104(7):2032-9.
38. Bray D, Henstrom DK, Cheney ML, et al. Assessing outcomes in facial reanimation: evaluation and validation of the SMILE system for measuring lip excursion during smiling. Arch Facial Plast Surg. 2010;12(5):352-4.
39. Hadlock T. Facial paralysis: research and future directions. Facial Plast Surg. 2008;24(2)260-7.
40. Hadlock T, Sundback C. Biologically inspired approaches to drug delivery for nerve regeneration. Expert Opin Biol Ther. 2006;6:1105-11.

7

Managing the Complications of Bariatric Surgery

Hamish Noble, Richard Welbourn

INTRODUCTION

The obesity epidemic and its associated diseases threaten to overwhelm global healthcare resources. More than 1 million adults in the UK have a body mass index (BMI) greater than 40.[1] By 2050, 60% of men, 50% of women and some 25% children under the age of 16 in the UK will be obese,[2] and the indirect costs to the National Health Service (NHS) of treating associated diabetes may have reached £50 billion per annum.

Bariatric surgery is the only intervention that gives long-standing improvement or resolution of obesity-related conditions and also survival benefit.[3,4] It is highly cost-effective.[5] Despite this, just 8,087 bariatric procedures were performed in the NHS in England in 2010-11.[6] In the US and some European countries, the number of operations performed has now surpassed cholecystectomy equivalent to more than 50,000 procedures annually in the UK. Data from the UK and Ireland National Bariatric Surgery Registry (NBSR)[7] indicate that in 2009-10, 67%, 21% and 10.5% of patients underwent laparoscopic Roux-en-Y gastric bypass (LRYGB), laparoscopic adjustable gastric band (LAGB) and sleeve gastrectomy (SG), respectively.

The number of bariatric operations is likely to increase for the foreseeable future. It is essential that the non-bariatric general gastrointestinal surgeon has an understanding of the anatomical arrangements of these operations (Figs 7.1A to C) and their common complications. Here, we provide an update and overview for trainees approaching their surgical examinations and for non-specialists focussing on these procedures.

RISK, RISK REDUCTION AND IMPROVING OUTCOMES

Data from the US[8] and the UK[7] clearly show that the prevalence of obesity-related co-morbid conditions, such as hypertension, diabetes, hyperlipidaemia, heart failure, asthma, obstructive sleep apnoea, functional impairment, pulmonary hypertension, deep vein thrombosis/pulmonary embolism (DVT/PE) risk and venous ulceration all increase rapidly with increasing BMI. Data from the NBSR[7] demonstrate that 16%, 37%, 47% and 54% of those with a BMI less than 40, 40–49.9, 50–59.9 and greater

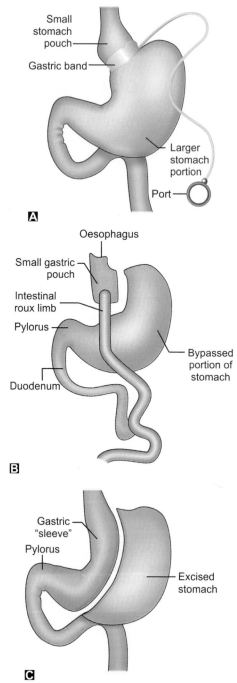

Figures 7.1A to C: Anatomy of (A) laparoscopic adjustable gastric band (LAGB), (B) Laparoscopic Roux-en-Y gastric bypass (LRYGB) and (C) sleeve gastrectomy (SG)

Source: Reproduced with permission from Ethicon Endo-Surgery

than 60, respectively have at least four obesity-related co-morbidities. Thus, surgery in the morbidly obese is inherently risky, and that risk needs to be minimised.

The Obesity Surgery Mortality Risk Score[9] was developed to stratify expected mortality for LRYGB and identified age (> 45 years), male sex, BMI greater than 50, hypertension and risk of DVT/PE as being predictive factors. Those with 4–5 factors have a 12-fold increase of mortality (2.4%) compared to those with less than or equal to one factor (0.2%). Two factors, male sex and hypertension, are associated with central obesity and present technically more challenging operations. Thus, 'liver shrinkage' diets[10] should be used routinely for at least 2 weeks preoperatively to reduce the risk of complications, and more weight loss may be mandated if there is a 'hard' abdomen in central obesity.

All patients should be assessed preoperatively by a multidisciplinary team, whose members may include a bariatric physician, dietician, specialist nurse, surgeon, anaesthetist and a psychologist.[11-14] This approach allows the optimisation of medical treatment of co-morbid conditions and the diagnosis and treatment of occult disease such as sleep apnoea. Attendance at preoperative education sessions also helps to ensure patients are fully supported, engaged and motivated.

There is a long learning curve for laparoscopic bariatric surgery, particularly LRYGB, with increased rates of complications during this time.[15] It is accepted that the learning curve for LRYGB is approximately 100 cases, which can be shortened with mentorship or within a fellowship programme.[16,17] The safety of bariatric surgery is known to be superior in high-surgeon and high-hospital volume centres,[18-20] and Centres of Excellence programmes have rightly pushed the need for specialisation.

Data from the national databases and registries of the NBSR,[7] hospital episode statistics data,[21] longitudinal assessment of bariatric surgery[22] and the American College of Surgeons Bariatric Surgical Center Network[23] have quantified risk of mortality and 30-day reoperation rates in large numbers of patients. In hospital, mortality for LAGB, SG and LRYGB have been shown to be approximately 0.05–0.1%, 0.1% and 0.2%, respectively. Thirty-day reoperation rates were approximately 0.9%, 3% and 4.5%, respectively.

> **Key Point**
>
> Bariatric surgery, including gastric banding, should be performed in high-volume centres in order to minimise operative risk and optimise long-term outcomes. The learning curve is shortened within a fellowship programme and with mentorship.

COMPLICATIONS OF GASTRIC BANDING

Laparoscopic adjustable gastric band has the lowest perioperative morbidity and mortality of current bariatric operations. However, it is estimated that

10–20% of patients will require reoperation over 5–10 years, with one study showing a 21% reoperation rate over 7 years.[24]

Early

Dysphagia

The most common immediate postoperative complication is an acutely obstructed band due to oedema, haematoma or failure to reflect a large oesophageal fat pad off the cardia (particularly in men with a higher BMI). This is usually self-limiting, but urgent band de-filling may relieve the problem if it was filled at the time of surgery.

Port Infection

Infection at the access port is disastrous (Fig. 7.2). Prophylactic antibiotics should be administered preoperatively. If infection occurs, a pragmatic approach in the first instance is a prolonged course of antibiotics. Some have used gentamicin impregnated beads placed around the port with success.[25] Ultimately, the port may have to be removed leaving the band in place. A new access port may then be reimplanted and reconnected once the sepsis has resolved.

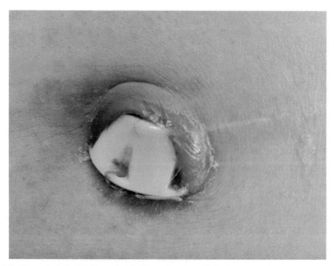

Figure 7.2: Grossly infected band access port extruding through the skin from its point of fixation on the anterior abdominal wall

Late

Band Slip

The incidence of slippage or herniation of the stomach up through the band varies in the literature due to the lack of definition (Fig. 7.3). It is reported

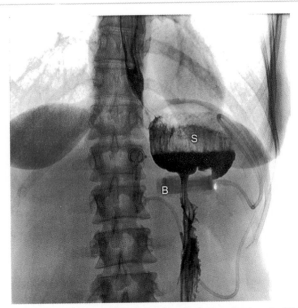

Figure 7.3: Contrast swallow of slipped gastric band. Note the band's (B) horizontal position with prolapse of the fundus of the stomach (S) through the band

in 1–20% of patients.[26] Slippage typically occurs after 2–3 years but can happen early particularly when gastro-gastric sutures have not been used.[27] Ninety-five percent of bands within the NBSR are sutured.[7] Most slippages are chronic and present with loss of restriction, reflux, pain and vomiting. If suspected, bands should be de-filled for a period, which may resolve symptoms but most will require revision and repositioning.

Acute slippage with strangulation of herniated stomach is an emergency, which presents with pain and dysphagia (Fig. 7.4). Treatment consists of de-filling the band with a non-coring Huber needle immediately on arrival in hospital (Figs 7.5 and 7.6). On a plain abdominal radiograph, the axis of a well-positioned band points towards the left shoulder, whereas a slipped band tends to lie horizontally or even point towards the left iliac fossa. Diagnosis is confirmed by water-soluble contrast swallow demonstrating herniation of the stomach up through the band with little or no passage of contrast through the stoma. If de-filling of the band produces prompt relief, this may be all that is needed acutely. However, if pain continues, i.e. there is suspicion of ongoing gastric ischaemia, then laparoscopy to remove, undo or reposition the band should be undertaken without delay.

Symmetric Pouch Dilatation

Symmetric or concentric dilatation of the proximal gastric pouch is recognised as a separate entity from slippage occurring in 4.4% of patients in one series (Fig. 7.7). This is not an emergency and presents with loss of restriction and reflux. It is thought to occur from excessive pressure within

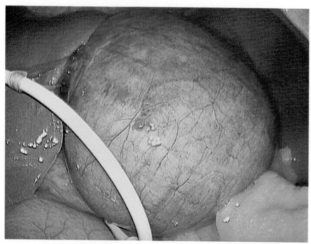

Figure 7.4: An acute band slippage with herniation of strangulated stomach up through the band. A fluid level is seen in the stomach

Courtesy: John Dixon, Melbourne

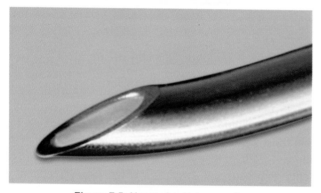

Figure 7.5: Non-coring Huber needle

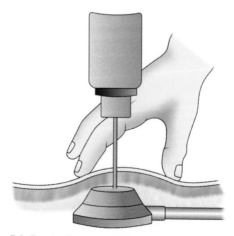

Figure 7.6: Band adjustment via access port with Huber needle

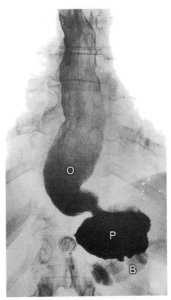

Figure 7.7: Symmetrical pouch dilatation after laparoscopic Roux-en-Y gastric bypass (LRYGB). Note the capacious gastric pouch (P) with an associated dilated oesophagus (O). The band (B) is correctly positioned

the pouch due to a combination of eating too much too quickly and an overlying inflated band.[28] Again, de-filling of the band and re-education of eating habits may help, but many will need the band repositioning higher on the stomach with a new posterior gastric tunnel.

> **Key Point**
>
> Any patient with a gastric band who presents as an emergency with upper abdominal pain and dysphagia should be considered to have an acute band slippage until proven otherwise. This requires urgent band de-filling to prevent gastric ischaemia, and every emergency department and admitting surgical ward should have Huber needles available and teams trained to do this.

Megaoesophagus

Gross dilatation of the oesophagus with oesophageal dysmotility occurs in approximately 1%[29] causing loss of restriction, reflux and regurgitation (Fig. 7.8). The mechanisms are not fully understood but migration of the band up onto the gastro-oesophageal junction with loss of the normal satiety feedback may be involved. Treatment is as for symmetric pouch dilatation.

Band Erosion

Erosion (Fig. 7.9) may be asymptomatic but often presents simply with sudden loss of restriction. Occasionally, migratory infection present at the access port can be the only sign (Fig. 7.10). In a recent systematic review, the risk of erosion was 1.4–10% depending on operative technique (perigastric > pars flaccida) and surgeon experience.[30] Diagnosis is usually made at

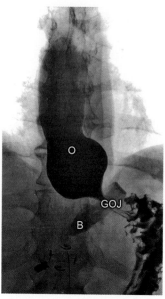

Figure 7.8: Megaoesophagus after laparoscopic Roux-en-Y gastric bypass (LRYGB). A grossly dilated oesophagus (O) above a malpositioned band (B) placed at the gastro-oesophageal junction (GOJ) rather than around the cardia

endoscopy or contrast swallow. Removal of the band may be performed endoscopically with a wire loop cutter or laparoscopically[31] with removal of the band through a gastrotomy some distance away from the band with repair and drainage to the stomach.

Port and Tubing Problems

Approximately, half of band reoperations are due to problems with the access port or tubing.[32] Typical band 'service' problems include tubing puncture and leak close to the port from a Huber needle, tubing fracture, disconnection and tilting of the access port preventing adjustments.

> **Key Point**
>
> Upto 10–20% of patients may require reoperation over 5–10 years after LAGB.

COMPLICATIONS OF ROUX-EN-Y GASTRIC BYPASS

Early

Anastomotic Leak

Anastomotic leak is the most feared complication and occurs in upto 3%.[33] Commonly, leaks happen at the gastro-jejunal anastomosis or on the gastric pouch (58%) with most others on the gastric remnant (25%) or at the jejuno-jejunal anastomosis (9%).[34] Due to the enhanced recovery of these

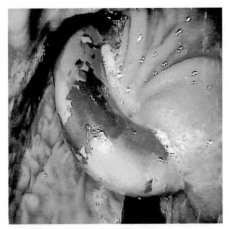

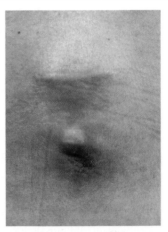

Figure 7.9: Endoscopic retroflexed view showing complete band erosion through the wall of the stomach

Fig. 7.10: Cellulitis around the band access port indicating late infection +/- band erosion

patients, who are allowed to drink on returning to the ward, a leak from the gastro-jejunal anastomosis will usually present within 24 hours. Leaks from the jejuno-jejunal anastomosis tend to present later, typically after 4–5 days. Any patient with a persistent tachycardia, temperature or feeling of impending doom should be considered to have a leak until proven otherwise. Laboratory tests may be falsely reassuring as may a normal pulse, since many are on beta-blockers. Contrast computed tomography (CT) may help but a very low threshold for same day laparoscopy is best. As a rule, patients should look completely well at 24 hours after LRYGB or SG, and if not, they should be considered for urgent investigation with a low threshold for re-laparoscopy.

Treatment should be aimed at early repair if possible, but most importantly drainage and creation of a controlled fistula if direct repair is not achievable. A feeding jejunostomy may be a valuable lifeline as healing is invariably prolonged during the catabolic period of rapid weight loss. Any evidence of obstruction distal to the leak should be sought and rectified. Self-expanding double covered stents have been used for leaks from the gastric pouch, which fail to heal with these measures.[35]

> **Key Point**
>
> Early recognition and treatment of anastomotic leaks in bariatric surgery is essential to prevent mortality. Any patient unwell after 24 hours needs urgent investigations, with a low threshold for re-laparoscopy .

Staple Line Bleeding

Bleeding from staple lines may be intraluminal, presenting with haematemesis and melaena, or extraluminal and occult. It has been reported in upto 4% following bypass.[36] The majority will settle. Some may need blood transfusion; clotting abnormalities should be corrected and proton pump inhibitors should be given. Endoscopic haemostasis is usually successful for proximal bleeding, which does not resolve and reoperation is rarely needed. The use of a circular stapler for the gastro-jejunal anastomosis is associated with more bleeding than linear stapled or hand sewn techniques.[37]

Late

Obstruction

The incidence of small bowel obstruction with LRYGB is approximately 4.4%. It usually occurs after 1–2 years, which coincides with maximum weight loss.[38] Half of cases are internal hernias[39] with most others due to adhesions, abdominal wall hernias or anastomotic strictures (see below). The anatomical arrangement following LRYGB leaves two or three mesenteric defects depending on whether the Roux limb has been taken in an antecolic or retrocolic route: (1) at the jejuno-jejunal anastomosis, (2) Petersen's defect posterior to the Roux limb as it passes through the mesocolon or over the colon, and (3) the mesocolic window in the retrocolic route (Fig. 7.11). The frequency of internal herniation may be influenced by the route of the Roux limb (possibly less with the antecolic route)[39] and whether or not mesenteric defects were closed at operation. Data from the NBSR suggest that only 30% of defects are currently closed.[7] An ongoing randomised controlled trial (RCT) from the Scandinavian Obesity Surgery Registry (SOReg) (Ingmar Näslund, personal communication) will provide a better level of evidence as to whether mesenteric defects should be closed routinely.

Obstruction at the jejuno-jejunostomy can present as closed loop obstruction (Fig. 7.12) of the gastric remnant, therefore, may be life-threatening. More usually, obstruction here presents insidiously with left upper quadrant pain after eating. A contrast CT is usually diagnostic. Laparoscopic reduction of hernias and inspection and closure of all defects with a nonabsorbable suture should be possible in most cases.

Paraumbilical hernias are extremely common in bariatric patients. If present at the time of the initial bariatric operation, they can either be repaired or left completely alone with omentum within them, to be fixed once weight loss has been achieved. Removing the omentum and exposing the defect inevitably leads to postoperative small bowel obstruction.

> **Key Point**
>
> General surgeons need to have a high index of suspicion for an internal hernia in a bypass patient presenting as an emergency with unexplained abdominal pain.

Anastomotic Stricture

A variety of techniques are used to form the pouch-jejunal anastomosis with stricturing reported in approximately 5%.[40] Strictures tend to occur

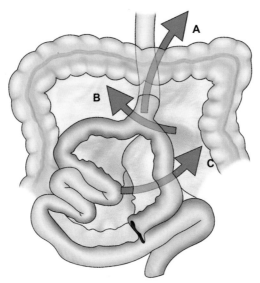

Figure 7. 11: Mesenteric defects following laparoscopic Roux-en-Y gastric bypass (LRYGB). Note the (A) Mesocolic defect—alongside the Roux limb in the retrocolic tunnel (B) Petersen's defect—underneath the Roux limb as it passes behind the transverse colon (C) Jejuno-jejunal—underneath the jejuno-jejunal anastomosis

Source: Schweitzer MA, DeMaria EJ, Broderick TH, et al. Laparoscopic closure of mesenteric defects after Roux-en-Y gastric bypass. J Laparoendosc Adv Surg Tech A. 2000;10:173-5.

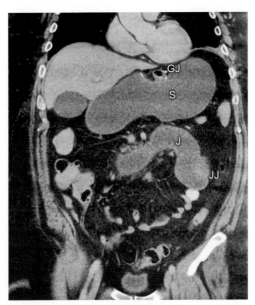

Figure 7.12: Closed loop obstruction at the jejuno-jejunostomy (JJ) after laparoscopic Roux-en-Y gastric bypass (LRYGB). Note the dilated proximal jejunum (J) and remnant stomach (S). The gastro-jejunal anastomosis is also seen (GJ)

soon after surgery and respond well to endoscopic balloon dilatation. In one report, circular stapled anastomoses with a 21 mm diameter stapler gave stricture rates of around 15% but this was significantly reduced by using a 25 mm stapler.[41] A recent analysis of a large series comparing stricture rates with hand sewn, linear stapler and 25 mm circular stapled techniques did not show any difference.[42]

Marginal Ulcers

Ulceration at the gastro-jejunal anastomosis usually presents in the first few months with pain and vomiting in upto 15% of patients.[43] It usually responds to proton pump inhibitors and eradication of *Helicobacter pylori*, if present, which many surgeons do prophylactically. The exact mechanisms involved are poorly understood. Non-healing is associated with a longer gastric pouch (more parietal tissue for acid production), smoking, nonsteroidal anti-inflammatories and the presence of a gastro-gastric fistula.[43,44] Revisional surgery is usually only required in rare (1%) cases of fistulation.[45]

COMPLICATIONS OF SLEEVE GASTRECTOMY

Early

Staple Line Leak and Bleeding

The American Society for Metabolic and Bariatric Surgery (ASMBS) position statement on SG suggests a leak rate of 2.2% and significant bleed rate of 1.2%.[46] In an effort to reduce staple line complications, most surgeons will use reinforcement with either buttressing material or oversewing. Some evidence suggests that reinforcement might reduce bleeding[47] but it does not reduce leaks.[48] However, leaks may be reduced by using larger (40 Fr) bougies to size the tube.[48] Recently, data from a large registry of 1,324 patients in Germany had similar results with leaks in 2.5% and bleeding in 2%. In this series, 90% of staple lines were either buttressed or oversewn.[49]

Leaks from the gastric tube occur in the proximal third of the stomach in 89%.[48] Stapling too close to the angle of His, the relative back pressure caused by the pylorus and the relative thinness of the proximal stomach are thought to be responsible. As with anastomotic leaks after LRYGB, they may take months to heal and the mainstay of treatment is early diagnosis, reoperation and drainage. Self-expanding stents may also help, particularly, if there is any narrowing of the sleeve distal to the leak.[35]

> **Key Point**
>
> Staple line complications following sleeve gastrectomy may be reduced by buttressing or oversewing with an absorbable suture.

Late

Reflux

In contrast to LRYGB, which has an additional benefit of being a very effective treatment for gastro-oesophageal reflux in the morbidly obese,[50] there is some emerging evidence that SG is associated with increased symptomatic reflux postoperatively.[51,52] Therefore, most agree that any crural defect should be sought and repaired at the time of surgery.

Stricture

The gastric sleeve is usually fashioned over a small 32–34 Ch bougie to minimise the gastric reservoir and ensure adequate weight loss. The stricture rate in the ASMBS review was 0.6%.[46] Strictures will usually respond to endoscopic dilatation or stenting. Patients whose strictures fail to resolve may be best served by conversion to another bariatric procedure such as LRYGB or duodenal switch.

NUTRITIONAL CONSEQUENCES OF BARIATRIC SURGERY

Consensus guidelines issued by the American Association of Clinical Endocrinologists, The Obesity Society and ASMBS describe the essential lifelong monitoring and supplementation of vitamins and minerals that is recommended for all patients,[11] noting particularly that in any case the obese state predisposes to vitamin deficiency. In LRYGB, the absorption of calcium, iron, vitamin B_{12}, folate and thiamine is impaired due to food bypassing the duodenum and proximal jejunum.

All patients having bariatric surgery should take multivitamins, calcium and vitamin D, iron (menstruating women) and vitamin B_{12} (from 6 months postoperatively). Blood indices should be monitored every 3 months for the first year and then yearly thereafter.

Nutritional deficiency is more common after biliopancreatic diversion (BPD) and its variant, duodenal switch (DS) with SG, which have short common channels resulting in significant protein and fat malabsorption. In addition to the rationale above, these patients need to be monitored for liver failure in the first few months following surgery; follow a high protein diet (80–120 g per day) and take increased supplementation of fat soluble vitamins.

> **Key Point**
>
> All patients require lifelong vitamin and mineral supplementation with monitoring of blood indices after bariatric surgery. This should be provided by a bariatric physician, specialist nurse or general practitioner with a specialist interest.

THROMBOEMBOLIC COMPLICATIONS

Fatal pulmonary embolism accounts for half of all deaths after LRYGB with an incidence of 0.1%.[53] Thromboembolic disease in bariatric patients is associated with male sex, age, BMI, surgery lasting more than 3 hours and the more complex procedures of LRYGB and BPD.[54] Routine use of thromboembolic deterrent (TED) stockings and pneumatic calf compression intraoperatively is imperative. Most now prescribe a course of low molecular weight heparin for at least 1 week after surgery. Inferior cava filters may be considered in very high-risk patients but there is little evidence for their efficacy in this group.

GALLSTONES/BILE DUCT STONES

Gallstones have been shown to develop in approximately 30% of patients during the first 6 months following open gastric bypass when weight loss is most profound.[55] Currently, there is no consensus as to whether patients having malabsorptive procedures should undergo prophylactic cholecystectomy at the same time. Recent data from a large population-based study has shown a 5-fold increase in cholecystectomy following LRYGB but noted a degree of selection bias, and the authors advocated an expectant policy.[56] An alternative approach is to prescribe ursodeoxycholic acid during the phase of rapid weight loss as this reduces gallstone formation but it is expensive and there can be poor compliance due to side effects.[55] Most surgeons only perform concurrent cholecystectomy in symptomatic patients with 4.9% of LRYGB patients undergoing cholecystectomy at their index operation currently in the UK.[7]

Access to the bile duct via endoscopic retrograde cholangiopancreatography (ERCP) following LRYGB, BPD or DS is limited. Bile duct stones presenting in these patients present a particular challenge for which there are three main options: (1) laparoscopic bile

Key Points

1. Bariatric surgery, including gastric banding, should be performed in high-volume centres in order to minimise operative risk and optimise long-term outcomes. The learning curve is shortened within a fellowship programme and with mentorship.

2. Any patient with a gastric band who presents as an emergency with upper abdominal pain and dysphagia should be considered to have an acute band slippage until proven otherwise. This requires urgent band de-filling to prevent gastric ischaemia, and every emergency department and admitting surgical ward should have Huber needles available and teams trained to do this.

3. Upto 10–20% of patients may require reoperation over 5–10 years after LAGB.

4. Early recognition and treatment of anastomotic leaks in bariatric surgery is essential to prevent mortality. Any patient unwell after 24 hours needs urgent investigations considered with a low threshold for re-laparoscopy.

5. General surgeons need to have a high index of suspicion for an internal hernia in a bypass patient presenting as an emergency with unexplained abdominal pain.

6. Staple line complications following sleeve gastrectomy may be reduced by buttressing or oversewing with an absorbable suture.

7. All patients require life-long vitamin and mineral supplementation with monitoring of blood indices after bariatric surgery. This should be provided by a bariatric physician, specialist nurse or general practitioner with a specialist interest.

duct exploration during cholecystectomy, (2) ERCP facilitated by a double balloon enteroscopy technique or (3) laparoscopic-assisted transgastric ERCP. In view of this it is recommended that consideration should be made to performing an intraoperative cholangiogram on all patients who undergo cholecystectomy after these procedures.

SUMMARY

The perfect bariatric operation would have low mortality and morbidity, achieve 100% excess weight loss, reverse all obesity-related co-morbidity, does not require revision/reoperation and have minimal long-term consequences. None exists, which explains the variety of procedures currently undertaken. At present, the type of operation performed is largely governed by patient choice, surgeon bias and local expertise, as there is very limited randomised evidence.

There are overwhelming data to show that bariatric surgery should be performed in high-volume centres by teams experienced in the management of these challenging patients so as to minimise complications. However, in view of the rapid increase in the numbers of operations carried out, it is essential that all gastrointestinal surgeons understand the common potential postoperative problems, which may well present locally.

REFERENCES

1. National Obesity Observatory. Available from www.noo.org.uk [Accessed August, 2012].
2. Department of Health. Foresight. (2007). Tackling Obesities: Future Choices—Project. [online] Available from http://webarchive.nationalarchives.gov.uk/+/www.dh.gov.uk/en/Publichealth/Healthimprovement/Obesity/DH_079713 [Accessed August, 2012]
3. Sjöström L, Narbro K, Sjöström CD, et al. Effects of bariatric surgery on mortality in Swedish obese subjects. N Engl J Med. 2007;357:741-52.
4. Colquitt JL, Picot J, Loveman E, et al. Surgery for obesity. Cochrane Database Syst Rev. 2009; (2):CD003641.
5. Picot J, Jones J, Colquitt JL, et al. The clinical effectiveness and cost-effectiveness of bariatric (weight loss) surgery for obesity: a systematic review and economic evaluation. Health Technol Assess. 2009;13(41):1-190, 215-357, iii-iv. Review.
6. The NHS Information Centre. (2012). Statistics on obesity, physical activity and diet: England, 2012. [online] Available from http://www.aso.org.uk/wp-content/uploads/downloads/2012/03/2012-Statistics-on-Obesity-Physical-Activity-and-Diet-England.pdf [Accessed August, 2012].
7. Welbourn R, Fiennes A, Kinsman R, et al. The National Bariatric Surgery Registry: First Registry Report to March 2010. Dendrite Clinical Systems 2011. ISBN: 1-903968-27-5.
8. LABS Writing Group for the LABS Consortium, Belle SH, Chapman W, et al. Relationship of body mass index with demographic and clinical characteristics in the longitudinal assessment of bariatric surgery (LABS). Surg Obes Relat Dis. 2008;4(4):474-80.

9. DeMaria EJ, Murr M, Byrne TK, et al. Validation of the obesity surgery mortality risk score in a multicenter study proves it stratifies mortality risk in patients undergoing gastric bypass for morbid obesity. Ann Surg. 2007;246:578-82.

10. Fris RJ. Preoperative low energy diet diminishes liver size. Obes Surg. 2004;14(9):1165-70.

11. Mechanick JI, Kushner RF, Sugerman HJ, et al. AACE/TOS/ASMBS guidelines for clinical practice for the perioperative nutritional, metabolic and nonsurgical support of the bariatric surgery patient. Endocr Pract. 2008;14:S1-83.

12. National Institute for Health and Clinical Excellence. (2006). Obesity: the prevention, identification, assessment and management of overweight and obesity in adults and children. CG 43. [online] Available from http://www.nice.org.uk/CG43 [Accessed August, 2012].

13. McMahon MM, Sarr MG, Clark MM, et al. Clinical management after bariatric surgery: value of a multidisciplinary approach. Mayo Clin Proc. 2006;81:S34-45.

14. Kelly JJ, Shikora S, Jones DB, et al. Best practice updates for surgical care in weight loss surgery. Obesity. 2009;17(5):863-70.

15. Pournaras DJ, Jafferbhoy S, Titcomb DR, et al. Three hundred laparoscopic Roux-en-Y gastric bypasses: managing the learning curve in higher risk patients. Obes Surg. 2010;20(3):290-4.

16. Schirmer BD, Schauer PR, Flum DR, et al. Bariatric surgery training: getting your ticket punched. J Gastointest Surg. 2007;11:807-12.

17. Ballantyne GH, Ewing D, Capella RF, et al. The learning curve measured by operating times for laparoscopic and open gastric bypass: roles of surgeon's experience, institutional experience, body mass index and fellowship training. Obes Surg. 2005;15:172-82.

18. Courcoulas A, Schuchert M, Gatti G, et al. The relationship of surgeon and hospital volume to outcome after gastric bypass surgery in Pennsylvania: a 3-year summary. Surgery. 2003;134(4):613-21.

19. Flum DR, Dellinger EP. Impact of gastric bypass operation on survival: a population-based analysis. J Am Coll Surg. 2004;199:543-51.

20. Smith MD, Patterson E, Wahed AS, et al. Relationship between surgeon volume and adverse outcomes after LRYGB in Longitudinal Assessment of Bariatric Surgery (LABS) study. Surg Obes Relat Dis. 2010;6(2):118-25.

21. Burns EM, Naseem H, Bottle A, et al. Introduction of laparoscopic bariatric surgery in England: observational population cohort study. BMJ. 2010;341:c4296.

22. Flum D, Belle SH, King WC, et al. Perioperative safety in the longitudinal assessment of bariatric surgery. The Longitudinal Assessment of Bariatric Surgery (LABS) Consortium. N Engl J Med. 2009;361:445-54.

23. Hutter MM, Schirmer BD, Jones DB, et al. First report from the American College of Surgeons Bariatric Surgery Center Network: laparoscopic sleeve gastrectomy has morbidity and effectiveness positioned between the band and the Bypass. Ann Surg. 2011;254:410-22.

24. Suter M, Calmes JM, Paroz A, et al. A 10-year experience with laparoscopic gastric banding for morbid obesity: high long-term complication and failure rates. Obes Surg. 2006;16:829-35.

25. Speybrouck S, Aelvoet C, Tollens T, et al. Use of gentamicin in the treatment of access-port infections. Obes Surg. 2005;15(9):1278-81.

26. Egan RJ, Monkhouse SJ, Meredith HE, et al. The reporting of gastric band slip and related complications: a review of the literature. Obes Surg. 2011;21(8):1280-8.

27. Lazzati A, Polliand C, Porta M, et al. Is fixation during gastric banding necessary? A randomised clinical study. Obes Surg. 2011;21(12):1859-63.

28. Brown WA, Burton PR, Anderson M, et al. Symmetrical pouch dilatation after laparoscopic adjustable gastric banding: incidence and management. Obes Surg. 2008;18(9):1104-8.

29. Arias IE, Radulescu M, Stiegeler R, et al. Diagnosis and treatment of megaesophagus after adjustable gastric banding for morbid obesity. Surg Obes Relat Dis. 2009;5(2):156-9.

30. Egberts K, Brown WA, O'Brien PE. Systematic review of erosion after laparoscopic adjustable gastric banding. Obes Surg. 2011;21(8):1272-9.

31. Abu-Abeid S, Szold A. Laparoscopic management of Lap-Band erosion. Obes Surg. 2001;11:87-9.

32. Tog CH, Halliday J, Khor Y, et al. Evolving pattern of laparoscopic gastric band access port complications. Obes Surg. 2012;22(6):863-5.

33. Lee S, Carmody B, Wolfe L, et al. Effect of location and speed of diagnosis on anastomotic leak outcomes in 3828 gastric bypass cases. J Gastrointest Surg. 2007;11:708-13.

34. Gonzalez R, Sarr MG, Smith CD, et al. Diagnosis and contemporary management of anastomotic leaks after gastric bypass for obesity. J Am Coll Surg. 2007;204:47-55.

35. Eubanks S, Edwards CA, Fearing NM, et al. Use of endoscopic stents to treat anastomotic complications after bariatric surgery. J Am Coll Surg. 2008;206(5):935-8; discussion 938-9.

36. Nguyen NT, Longoria M, Chalifoux S, et al. Gastrointestinal hemorrhage after laparoscopic gastric bypass. Obes Surg. 2004;14:1308-12.

37. Finks JF, Carlin A, Share D, et al. Effect of surgical techniques on clinical outcomes after laparoscopic gastric bypass—results from the Michigan Bariatric Surgery Collaborative. Surg Obes Relat Dis. 2011;7(3):284-9.

38. Husain S, Ahmed AR, Johnson J, et al. Small-bowel obstruction after laparoscopic Roux-en-Y gastric bypass: etiology, diagnosis and management. Arch Surg. 2007;142(10):988-93.

39. Ahmed AR, Rickards G, Husain S, et al. Trends in internal hernia incidence after Laparoscopic Roux-en-Y gastric bypass. Obes Surg. 2007;17:1563-6.

40. Higa K, Ho T, Tercero F, et al. Laparoscopic Roux-en-Y gastric bypass: 10-year follow-up. Surg Obes Relat Dis. 2011;7(4):516-25.

41. Gould JC, Garren M, Boll V, et al. The impact of circular stapler diameter on the incidence of gastrojejunostomy stenosis and weight loss following laparoscopic Roux-en-Y gastric bypass. Surg Endosc. 2006;20(7):1017-20.

42. Bendewald FP, Choi JN, Blythe LS, et al. Comparison of hand-sewn, linear-stapled, and circular-stapled gastrojejunostomy in laparoscopic Roux-en-Y gastric bypass. Obes Surg. 2011;21(11):1671-5.

43. Azagury DE, Abu Dayyeh BK, Greenwalt IT, et al. Marginal ulceration after laparoscopic Roux-en-Y gastric bypass surgery: characteristics, risk factors, treatment, and outcomes. Endoscopy. 2011;43(11):950-4.

44. El-Hayek K, Timratana P, Shimizu H, et al. Marginal ulcer after laparoscopic Roux-en-Y gastric bypass: what have we really learned? Surg Endosc. 2012 Apr 28 [Epub ahead of print].

45. Carrodeguas L, Szomstein S, Soto F, et al. Management of gastrogastric fistulas after divided laparoscopic Roux-en-Y gastric bypass surgery for morbid obesity: analysis of 1,292 consecutive patients and review of literature. Surg Obes Relat Dis. 2005;1(5):467-74.

46. American Society for Metabolic and Bariatric Surgery. (2011). Updated position statement on sleeve gastrectomy as a bariatric procedure. [online] Available from http://s3.amazonaws.com/publicASMBS/GuidelinesStatements/Position Statement/ASMBS-SLEEVE-STATEMENT-2011_10_28.pdf [Accessed August, 2012].

47. Dapri G, Cadière GB, Himpens J. Reinforcing the staple line during laparoscopic sleeve gastrectomy: prospective randomized clinical study comparing three different techniques. Obes Surg. 2010;20(4):462-7.

48. Aurora AR, Khaitan L, Saber AA. Sleeve gastrectomy and the risk of leak: a systematic analysis of 4,888 patients. Surg Endosc. 2012;26(6):1509-15.

49. Stroh C, Weiner R, Horbach T, et al. Results of Sleeve Gastrectomy in Germany—Data on Nationwide Survey on Quality Assurance in Bariatric Surgery in Germany. Surgical Science. 2012;3:169-76.

50. Nelson LG, Gonzalez R, Haines K, et al. Amelioration of gastroesophageal reflux symptoms following laparoscopic Roux-en-Y gastric bypass for clinically significant obesity. Am Surg. 2005;71(11):950-3; discussion 953-4.

51. Howard DD, Caban AM, Cendan JC, et al. Gastroesophageal reflux after sleeve gastrectomy in morbidly obese patients. Surg Obes Relat Dis. 2011;7(6):709-13.

52. Carter PR, LeBlanc KA, Hausmann MG, et al. Association between gastroesophageal reflux disease and laparoscopic sleeve gastrectomy. Surg Obes Relat Dis. 2011;7(5):569-72.

53. Podnos YD, Jimenez JC, Wilson SE, et al. Complications after laparoscopic gastric bypass: a review of 3464 cases. Arch Surg. 2003;138(9):957-61.

54. Finks JF, English WJ, Carlin AM, et al. Predicting risk for venous thromboembolism with bariatric surgery: results from the Michigan Bariatric Surgery Collaborative. Ann Surg. 2012;255(6):1100-4 [Epub ahead of print].

55. Sugerman HJ, Brewer WH, Shiffman ML, et al. A multicenter, placebo-controlled, randomized, double-blind, prospective trial of prophylactic ursodiol for the prevention of gallstone formation following gastric bypass-induced rapid weight loss [with discussion]. Am J Surg. 1995;169:91-7.

56. Plecka Östlund M, Wenger U, Mattsson F, et al. Population-based study of the need for cholecystectomy after obesity surgery. Br J Surg. 2012;99(6):864-9.

8 | Metastases from Colorectal Cancer

Robert P Jones, Declan FJ Dunne, Graeme J Poston

Ten years ago, a diagnosis of metastatic colorectal cancer was associated with a survival of less than 3% at 5 years.[1] A small minority of patients with liver-only metastatic disease were offered surgical resection, and these patients had a 30–50% chance of being alive after 5 years.[2] This stark contrast highlighted the potential survival benefits of resection in appropriate cases, and led to a revolution in the approach to metastatic colorectal disease. Instead of a terminal diagnosis, it was recognised that in certain situations resection could offer the chance of cure.

About 30% of patients with colorectal cancer will have metastatic disease at the time of presentation, and a further 20% will develop liver disease after the primary colorectal malignancy has been resected.[2] In 2012, 20% of these patients will be candidates for potentially curative liver surgery,[3] with 5-year survival after resection approaching 50%.[4-16] However, 65% who survive for 5 years will experience disease recurrence.[17] Growing evidence shows that those patients who have liver-only recurrence benefit from repeat resection, with a survival benefit similar to primary resection.[18,19] This strategy of repeat intervention offers a further sub-group of patients, who although not necessarily 'cured', having their disease converted into a surgically controlled chronic condition.

> **Key Point**
>
> Without surgery, there are very few long-term survivors with metastatic colorectal cancer. For those who undergo surgery, around 50% will be alive 5 years later.

DEFINING RESECTABILITY IN COLORECTAL LIVER METASTASES

Over the last decade, the surgical approach to colorectal liver metastases has undergone a paradigm shift, as understanding the definition of resectability has evolved. Previously, patients with synchronous disease, rectal primary, multiple diffuse metastases, metastases larger than 5 cm, disease-free interval of less than 1 year from the diagnosis of primary disease or a high serum carcinoembryonic antigen (CEA) were considered irresectable and suitable only for palliative treatment.[20] Modern surgical techniques and chemotherapeutic regimens mean none of these contraindications now hold true.

Resectability with curative intent is now defined as the ability to successfully remove all residual disease from the liver with clear surgical margins whilst leaving adequate disease-free liver.[21] Resections are now routinely performed with a mortality of less than 1%.[17] The border between resectable and unresectable disease is constantly evolving as good outcomes are demonstrated in subsets of patients who would previously have been considered untreatable. Current contraindications to resection can be grouped into two main categories—technical or oncological.

Technical contraindications to resection are related to the anatomical location of metastases, mainly due to close proximity to major vascular or biliary drainage structures. The boundaries of technical resectability have been extended by the development of techniques, such as total vascular exclusion and *ex vivo* resection, which offer hope for certain patients with involvement of major vessels.[22] Resection with a negative surgical margin of 1 cm (R0) was considered the gold standard, but in an era of effective modern chemotherapy, patients with R1 resection (macroscopically negative margin) have similar survival to those with R0 resections.[23] Adequate hepatic parenchyma must be left after resection to maintain liver function. A future liver remnant (FLR) of 25% is considered sufficient to avoid postoperative hepatic failure,[24] although patients with impaired hepatic function, including those with chemotherapy-induced liver damage, may require a larger FLR. The regenerative nature of liver parenchyma means that significant regrowth takes place after resection, and this unique feature means that planned sequenced two-stage procedures are feasible, with parenchymal regeneration between resections ensuring adequate FLR.[25] This regenerative capacity is manipulated further using preoperative portal vein embolization to induce reactive hypertrophy in the proposed FLR.[26]

Oncological contraindications to resection include unresectable extrahepatic malignancy, although resectable extrahepatic disease is no longer seen as a barrier to surgery. Ten years ago, any extrahepatic metastatic disease was considered a contraindication to liver resection. However, studies have now shown long-term survivors in selected groups of patients with resected extrahepatic disease. Survival after partial pneumonectomy for colorectal metastases is similar to that seen after liver resection, with most series quoting a 5-year survival in the order of 40–50%, with low operative morbidity and mortality.[21,27-29] Repeat resection of pulmonary metastases may also confer survival benefit, with 5-year survival of 42% reported after repeat resection.[22] Limited peritoneal and hepatic pedicle nodal disease is also potentially curable, with 5-year survival around 25% following resection.[30]

National Institute of Clinical Excellence (NICE) guidance in the UK now recommends that surgery for colorectal liver metastases should be considered if a patient is fit enough, and complete resection can be achieved leaving adequate FLR.[23] The guidance gave no absolute contraindications to surgery, but suggested that liver resection should not be carried out in the presence of:

1. Non-treatable primary tumour
2. Widespread pulmonary disease
3. Locoregional recurrence
4. Uncontrollable peritoneal disease
5. Extensive nodal disease, such as retroperitoneal or mediastinal lymph nodes
6. Bone or central nervous system (CNS) metastases.

> **Key Point**
>
> Many patients are now considered suitable for potentially curative liver resection for metastatic colorectal cancer. However, surgery is not appropriate for patients with irresectable extrahepatic disease.

THE IMPORTANCE OF SPECIALIST MULTIDISCIPLINARY TEAM INPUT IN THE MANAGEMENT OF METASTATIC COLORECTAL CANCER

The management of advanced metastatic colorectal cancer is complex, so it is vital that patients have their treatment managed by highly specialised surgeons and oncologists. The UK system of local colorectal multidisciplinary teams (MDTs) organised into cancer networks, with recognised referral pathways to supraregional specialist MDTs, is designed to facilitate this process. However, even within this system there remains concern that not all patients with liver-only metastatic disease are being reviewed by appropriate specialists. A 2010 UK population-based study of 114,155 patients who underwent primary colorectal cancer resection between 1998 and 2004 identified 3,116 (2.7%) patients who subsequently underwent resection for colorectal liver metastases, with the rate of hepatic resection varying widely between cancer networks (1.1–4.3%) and hospitals (0.7–6.8%) (Fig. 8.1).[24]

The authors suggested that inconsistent use of first-line chemotherapy and poor understanding of what is resectable disease may explain this variability, and argued that direct involvement of appropriate specialists was the only way to address these inequalities.

To help non-experts in decision making, a computer model (OncoSurge) was created to recommend optimal treatment strategies on a case-specific basis. An expert panel rated appropriateness of treatment (chemotherapy, resection or ablation) in 252 cases. A decision model was constructed, consensus measured and results validated using 48 virtual cases and 34 real cases with known outcomes. Consensus was achieved with overall agreement rates of 93.4–99.1%. This model combined the best available scientific evidence with the collective judgement of worldwide experts to yield a

> **Key Point**
>
> Metastatic colorectal cancer requires specialist management from expert surgeons and oncologists to ensure the best patient outcomes.

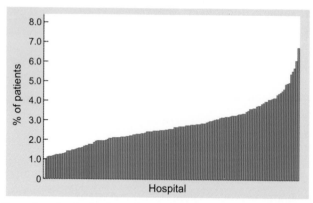

Figure 8.1: Proportion of patients who underwent liver resection within 3 years of diagnosis of colorectal cancer by National Health Service (NHS) hospital. The 700% variation in resection rates likely reflects non-specialist management of advanced colorectal cancer[24]

statement regarding the appropriateness of a particular treatment for each patient.

STAGING AND SELECTION OF PATIENTS FOR LIVER SURGERY

Patients with colorectal liver metastases must be fully staged prior to any treatment plan and this should be co-ordinated by a specialist MDT.[23] Computed tomography (CT) is now considered a standard of care for all patients with metastatic colorectal cancer.[23] Whilst CT remains the initial investigation of choice, it does have limitations including a high radiation dose and low sensitivity for the detection and characterisation of lesions smaller than 1 cm.

Magnetic resonance imaging (MRI) is a highly effective imaging modality for detecting and characterising liver lesions as it provides high lesion-to-liver contrast without using ionising radiation. Liver-specific contrast media are not taken up by colorectal hepatic metastases, so may aid in the characterisation of liver lesions that are either small or indeterminate using other imaging modalities.[31,32] Colorectal malignancies are often metabolically active and therefore have a greater glucose uptake relative to that of surrounding normal tissues. This can be identified with [^{18}F] fluoro-2-D-glucose positron emission tomography (FDG-PET). This modality is highly sensitive especially when combined with CT to allow accurate anatomical localisation (PET-CT).[25]

Traditionally, selection of patients for resection has focused on identifying patients with technically and oncologically resectable disease. There is now interest in identifying patients who have a higher operative risk, either because of reduced fitness or previously undetected cardiorespiratory co-morbidities. Cardiopulmonary exercise testing (CPET) has been shown to be a useful technique in quantifying this risk prior to major hepatobiliary surgery.[26]

TECHNICAL DEVELOPMENTS IN LIVER SURGERY

Recent innovations in liver surgery have focused on minimising blood loss during transection of the hepatic parenchyma. Inflow occlusion (Pringle manoeuvre) and low central venous pressure (CVP) anaesthesia aim to restrict blood flow through the liver but may result in an ischaemia reperfusion injury. There has therefore been an interest in parenchymal transection techniques that minimise blood loss. The most popular of these techniques include the ultrasonic aspirating dissector (CUSA), the hydrojet using a pressurised jet of water, the dissecting sealer (TissueLink) using radiofrequency energy and the Kelly-clamp crushing technique. These methods were compared in a randomised controlled trial,[33] which found no difference between the four techniques, although clamp crushing was associated with faster tissue transection.

There is increasing use of laparoscopic techniques in liver surgery. A recent meta-analysis[34] assessed 409 resections, of which 165 (40.3%) were laparoscopic and 244 (59.7%) were open. Operative blood loss and duration of hospital stay were significantly reduced after laparoscopic surgery with no difference in postoperative morbidity or medium-term oncological outcome.

> **Key Point**
>
> Technical developments aim to make surgery quicker and safer, as well as increasing the number of patients who can be offered surgery. Improved staging helps ensure that surgery is only performed in those patients in whom it is oncologically sensible.

ABLATIVE THERAPIES FOR COLORECTAL LIVER METASTASES

Ablative therapies aim to destroy tumour by the direct application of energy to disease. However, there remains a lack of clarity surrounding the precise role of ablation in the management of metastatic colorectal cancer. Recent American Society of Clinical Oncology (ASCO) guidelines[35] highlighted a wide variation in overall survival and local recurrence rates after ablation, and suggested that in the absence of adequate data, resection should remain the gold standard treatment for resectable disease. Despite these concerns, ablation still has a role as an adjunct to resection. Patients with small-volume resectable metastases who are not sufficiently fit to undergo liver resection should be considered for ablation as should those with limited liver metastases who have insufficient liver volume to undergo resection.

There is growing interest in the use of ablation alongside systemic chemotherapy for irresectable liver disease. Results of the EORTC 40004 (CLOCC) trial that compared systemic chemotherapy versus chemotherapy and radiofrequency ablation (RFA) for irresectable metastatic colorectal liver disease suggested a survival advantage for the combined arm.[36]

Radiofrequency ablation is the most widely used ablative technique and relies on direct current transmission through tissue to generate heat and cause an ablation. Increasing lesion size leads to exponential increases in resistance to current, limiting the size of the effective ablation zone and explaining the increased risk of local recurrence and diminished survival with lesions greater than 3 cm.[35] A meta-analysis of 95 published series reported a complication rate of 8.9%[37] and postoperative mortality rates between 0% and 0.5%, with a reported local recurrence rate of 10–31% which is much higher than the local recurrence rate reported after surgical resection with curative intent.[38] Microwave ablation has been designed to overcome some of the limitations of RFA and offers higher intratumoural temperatures, larger tumour ablation volumes and faster ablation times. Despite this, local recurrence after microwave ablation has been reported between 5% and 13%, with a major complication rate ranging from 3–16%.[38]

> **Key Point**
>
> Ablative therapies offer an alternative treatment for patients who cannot be resected. However, surgery remains the treatment of choice for resectable disease.

CHEMOTHERAPY FOR METASTATIC COLORECTAL CANCER

Chemotherapeutic manipulation of advanced colorectal cancer has undergone a paradigm shift over the last 15 years. Previously, patients with unresectable disease were treated solely with the aim of prolonging life. There is now growing recognition that some patients who may not be resectable at presentation become resectable after chemotherapy. This approach is often referred to as 'induction' or 'conversion' chemotherapy.[39]

By contrast, chemotherapy may be given during the perioperative period with the aim of reducing occult disease burden. This approach is referred to as 'true neoadjuvant' and 'adjuvant' therapy. Correct nomenclature is vitally important when it comes to explaining the intent of any chemotherapeutic regimen.

Conversion/Induction Chemotherapy

Resectability rates after chemotherapy for initially irresectable disease vary widely, with modern regimes achieving conversion rates approaching 60% (Fig. 8.2).[40] Attempting to bring unresectable disease to resection is worthwhile, with overall 5-year survival comparable between patients resectable at presentation and those converted to resectability after systemic chemotherapy.[41] Response to chemotherapy is known to correlate with resection rate,[40] and it seems sensible that patients with irresectable disease in

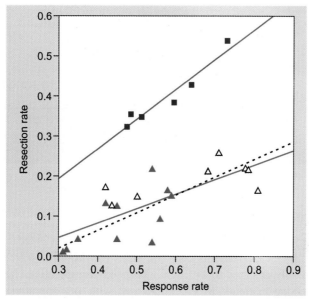

Figure 8.2: Rate of liver resection following systemic chemotherapy for initially unresectable disease. The solid squares represent patients with non-resectable metastases confined to the liver ('selected patients', r = 0.96, P = 0.002). Studies with non-selected patients with colorectal cancer are shown as triangles. Due to the high heterogeneity of these studies, the observed correlation is less strong (r = 0.74, P < 0.001, solid line). A similar correlation was observed when the phase III trials (filled triangles) were separately analysed (r = 0.67, P = 0.024, dashed line)[40]

the liver only should be treated with the most aggressive regimen possible to provide the greatest chance of being bought to potentially curative resection.

The UK NICE currently recommends the use of 5-FU, leucovorin and oxaliplatin-based regimens (FOLFOX) as first-line therapy for all patients with non-resectable disease, with irinotecan-based regimens (FOLFIRI) for second-line therapy after failure of first-line treatment. In liver-only irresectable disease, NICE guidance TA176 also recommends the use of the epidermal growth factor receptor (EGFR) monoclonal antibody, cetuximab, alongside FOLFOX as the first-line treatment for patients who are KRAS wild type (KRAS mutant tumours do not respond to this targeted therapy) (Fig. 8.3).

The CELIM study[42] assessed FOLFOX/FOLFIRI and cetuximab for a selected group of patients with unresectable metastatic liver-only disease in a randomised phase II study design and found response rates of 68% and 57%, respectively. Forty percent of the FOLFOX and cetuximab arm underwent resection compared to 43% of FOLFIRI and cetuximab. In a combined analysis of both arms, 67 patients with KRAS wild-type tumours achieved a response rate of 79%.

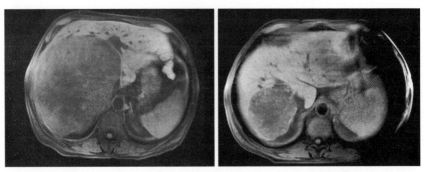

Figure 8.3: MRI scan of a patient with large colorectal liver metastasis, showing response to systemic FOLFOX chemotherapy with cetuximab

Perioperative Chemotherapy

The precise role of adjuvant and neoadjuvant chemotherapy in the management of resectable disease remains controversial. The EORTC 40983 phase III trial (commonly referred to as EPOC) assessed perioperative chemotherapy by randomising patients to chemotherapy with perioperative FOLFOX and surgery (six cycles before/after surgery) or surgery alone. Although often criticized, this study demonstrated a significantly improved 3-year progression free survival in the perioperative chemotherapy arm in resectable patients and remains the best available evidence supporting perioperative chemotherapy.[43] However, Adam et al[44] assessed 1,471 patients with solitary liver metastases, and compared those who underwent resection without chemotherapy and those treated with perioperative chemotherapy followed by resection. They found that preoperative chemotherapy had no impact on long-term outcome, but postoperative chemotherapy was associated with better overall and disease-free survival. A meta-analysis of trials assessing postoperative 5-FU-based chemotherapy demonstrated a trend towards improved disease-free and overall survival, but did not achieve statistical significance.[45]

Despite these controversies, expert consensus is that the majority of patients with colorectal liver disease should receive perioperative chemotherapy irrespective of their initial resectability,[46] with the rationale that this will result in the destruction of occult disease, allow a test of biology where progression despite chemotherapy signifies poor biology, as well as reduce lesion size improving resectability.

Chemotherapy-Associated Hepatotoxicity

Increased use of neoadjuvant treatment has resulted in a rise in chemotherapy-associated hepatotoxicity. Oxaliplatin is associated with sinusoidal obstructive syndrome, characterised by a tender, congested and dilated liver, whilst patients treated with irinotecan develop fatty infiltration and scarring (steatohepatitis).[47,48] Recognition of the growing number of patients coming to resection with chemotherapy-associated hepatotoxicity has led to growing interest in its impact on surgical outcome. The EORTC 40983 trial[43] comparing immediate surgery and perioperative FOLFOX demonstrated a higher rate of minor complications in the chemotherapy and surgery arm (25% vs 16%; p = 0.04). The MD Anderson group demonstrated an increased 90-day mortality in patients who had irinotecan-induced steatohepatitis compared to those who did not (14.7% vs 1.6%, p = 0.001).[47]

Postoperative morbidity does appear to be related to the duration of neoadjuvant chemotherapy. Karoui et al[49] demonstrated a higher morbidity in those patients who received more than six cycles (54% vs 19%, p = 0.047). However, this increased risk does appear to be reversible. Welsh et al[50] showed complication rates of 2.6%, 5.5% and 11% for patients with intervals of 9–12 weeks, 5–8 weeks and 4 weeks or less between cessation of chemotherapy and resection (p = 0.009).

Liver-Targeted Therapies

The unique blood supply of the liver, with portal flow supplying healthy hepatic parenchyma and arterial flow supplying metastatic disease has led to the concept of delivering therapy via the hepatic artery in an effort to increase metastatic exposure to the agent whilst reducing systemic dose and off-target side effects. A meta-analysis by Mocellin et al[51] found no evidence to support intra-arterial delivery instead of systemic chemotherapy in the treatment of irresectable colorectal metastases and so interest is now focused on the use of liver-targeted chemotherapy alongside systemic therapies to maximise response in liver dominant disease.

Adoption of hepatic arterial infusion (HAI), where a pump delivers therapy direct to a catheter placed in the hepatic artery, has been limited by high rates of technical complications with a reported 16% failure rate within 2 years of pump insertion.[52] Kemeny et al published an early phase I trial of 49 patients treated with systemic oxaliplatin alongside HAI floxuridine in irresectable liver-only disease. They reported 8% complete response rate, 84% partial response and 47% conversion to resectability, which increased to 57% in chemonaïve patients.[53,54] The same group recently reported their experience of adjuvant HAI alongside systemic FOLFOX/FOLFIRI in 125 resected patients, and reported improved overall and recurrence free survival.[55]

Drug eluting beads are compressible microspheres produced from polyvinyl alcohol (PVA) hydrogel loaded with drug (usually irinotecan). Doxorubicin-eluting bead transarterial chemoembolisation (DEB-TACE) offers a theoretical advantage over HAI of simplified delivery (embolisation and chemotherapy are combined). An international registry of 55 heavily pretreated patients treated with irinotecan beads demonstrated a response rate of 66% at 6 months, and 75% at 12 months. Median overall survival from time of first treatment was 19 months, with a progression free survival of 11 months. Six patients (10%) had their disease sufficiently downstaged to allow further treatment, with four undergoing resection and two undergoing RFA.[56]

Selective internal radiation therapy (SIRT) involves the delivery of radiation treatment by hepatic arterial administration of yttrium-90 (Y-90) microspheres. Y-90 is a high-energy, beta-particle-emitting isotope bound to resin microspheres, and the spheres are selectively delivered to tumour via intra-arterial embolisation. The randomised phase III FOXFIRE trial comparing systemic FOLFOX chemotherapy +/- SIRT for irresectable liver-only or liver-predominant disease is currently recruiting, and will help clarify the role of SIRT in the management of colorectal liver metastases.

> **Key Point**
>
> A combined surgical and oncological approach is essential for the treatment of metastatic colorectal cancer. Appropriate chemotherapy can bring patients with irresectable disease to potentially curative surgery.

CONCLUSIONS

Long-term survival for patients with colorectal liver metastases has improved enormously over the last 10 years with over 30% of all patients surviving more than 5 years after diagnosis, rising to over 60% if the liver disease is resectable. However, such outcomes can only be achieved within the setting of a multidisciplinary approach to management, with the liver surgeon key to the decision-making process.

> **Key Points**
>
> 1. Without surgery, there are very few long-term survivors with metastatic colorectal cancer. For those who undergo surgery, around 50% will be alive 5 years later.
> 2. Many patients are now considered suitable for potentially curative liver resection for metastatic colorectal cancer. However, surgery is not appropriate for patients with irresectable extrahepatic disease.
> 3. Metastatic colorectal cancer requires specialist management from expert surgeons and oncologists to ensure the best patient outcomes.
> 4. Technical developments aim to make surgery quicker and safer, as well as increasing the number of patients who can be offered surgery. Improved staging helps ensure that surgery is only performed in those patients in whom it is oncologically sensible.
> 5. Ablative therapies offer an alternative treatment for patients who cannot be resected. However, surgery remains the treatment of choice for resectable disease.
> 6. A combined surgical and oncological approach is essential for the treatment of metastatic colorectal cancer. Appropriate chemotherapy can bring patients with irresectable disease to potentially curative surgery.

REFERENCES

1. Rougier P, Milan C, Lazorthes F, et al. Prospective study of prognostic factors in patients with unresected hepatic meta-stases from colorectal cancer. Fondation Française de Cancérologie Digestive. Br J Surg. 1995;82(10):1397-400.

2. Scheele J, Stang R, Altendorf-Hofmann A, et al. Resection of colorectal liver metastases. World J Surg. 1995;19(1):59-71.

3. Adam R, Vinet E. Regional treatment of metastasis: surgery of colorectal liver metastases. Ann Oncol. 2004;15 Suppl 4:iv103-6.

4. Choti MA, Sitzmann JV, Tiburi MF, et al. Trends in long-term survival following liver resection for hepatic colorectal metastases. Ann Surg. 2002;235(6):759-66.

5. Nordlinger B, Vaillant JC, Guiguet M, et al. Survival benefit of repeat liver resections for recurrent colorectal metastases: 143 cases. Association Francaise de Chirurgie. J Clin Oncol. 1994;12(7):1491-6.

6. Yamada H, Kondo S, Okushiba S, et al. Analysis of predictive factors for recurrence after hepatectomy for colorectal liver metastases. World J Surg. 2001;25(9):1129-33.

7. Crowe PJ, Yang JL, Berney CR, et al. Genetic markers of survival and liver recurrence after resection of liver metastases from colorectal cancer. World J Surg. 2001;25(8):996-1001.

8. Mala T, Bøhler G, Mathisen, et al. Hepatic resection for colorectal metastases: can preoperative scoring predict patient outcome? World J Surg. 2002;26(11):1348-53.

9. Figueras J, Valls C, Rafecas A, et al. Resection rate and effect of postoperative chemotherapy on survival after surgery for colorectal liver metastases. Br J Surg. 2001;88(7):980-5.

10. Ambiru S, Miyazaki M, Isono T, et al. Hepatic resection for colorectal metastases: analysis of prognostic factors. Dis Colon Rectum. 1999;42(5):632-9.

11. Wang JY, Chiang JM, Jeng LB, et al. Resection of liver metastases from colorectal cancer: are there any truly significant clinical prognosticators? Dis Colon Rectum. 1996;39(8):847-51.

12. Rees M, Plant G, Bygrave S. Late results justify resection for multiple hepatic metastases from colorectal cancer. Br J Surg. 1997;84(8):1136-40.

13. Wanebo HJ, Chu QD, Vezeridis MP, et al. Patient selection for hepatic resection of colorectal metastases. Arch Surg. 1996;131(3):322-9.

14. Schlag P, Hohenberger P, Herfarth C. Resection of liver metastases in colorectal cancer: competitive analysis of treatment results in synchronous versus metachronous metastases. Eur J Surg Oncol. 1990;16(4):360-5.

15. Scheele J, Stangl R, Altendorf-Hofmann A, et al. Indicators of prognosis after hepatic resection for colorectal secondaries. Surgery. 1991;110(1):13-29.

16. Bakalakos EA, Burak WE, Young DC, et al. Is carcino-embryonic antigen useful in the follow-up management of patients with colorectal liver metastases? Am J Surg. 1999;177(1):2-6.

17. Mayo SC, Pawlik TM. Current management of colorectal hepatic metastasis. Expert Rev Gastroenterol Hepatol. 2009;3(2):131-44.

18. Adam R, Pascal G, Azoulay D, et al. Liver resection for colorectal metastases: the third hepatectomy. Ann Surg. 2003;238(6):871-83; discussion 883-4.

19. de Jong MC, Mayo SC, Pulitano C, et al. Repeat curative intent liver surgery is safe and effective for recurrent colorectal liver metastasis: results from an international multi-institutional analysis. J Gastrointest Surg. 2009;13(12):2141-51.

20. Poston GJ. Staging of advanced colorectal cancer. Surg Oncol Clin N Am. 2008;17(3):503-17, viii.

21. Pfannschmidt J, Muley T, Hoffmann H, et al. Prognostic factors and survival after complete resection of pulmonary metastases from colorectal carcinoma: experiences in 167 patients. J Thorac Cardiovasc Surg. 2003;126(3):732-9.

22. Kanzaki R, Higashiyama M, Oda K, et al. Outcome of surgical resection for recurrent pulmonary metastasis from colorectal carcinoma. Am J Surg. 2011;202(4):419-26.

23. Poston GJ, Tait D, O'Connell S, et al. Diagnosis and management of colorectal cancer: summary of NICE guidance. BMJ. 2011;343:d6751.
24. Morris EJ, Forman D, Thomas JD, et al. Surgical management and outcomes of colorectal cancer liver metastases. Br J Surg. 2010;97(7):1110-8.
25. Israel O, Mor M, Gaitini D, et al. Combined functional and structural evaluation of cancer patients with a hybrid camera-based PET/CT system using (18 F)-FDG. J Nucl Med. 2002;43(9):1129-36.
26. Snowden CP, Prentis JM, Anderson HL, et al. Submaximal cardiopulmonary exercise testing predicts complications and hospital length of stay in patients undergoing major elective surgery. Ann Surg. 2010;251(3):535-41.
27. Yedibela S, Klein P, Feuchter K, et al. Surgical management of pulmonary metastases from colorectal cancer in 153 patients. Ann Surg Oncol. 2006;13(11):1538-44.
28. Shiono S, Ishii G, Nagai K, et al. Predictive factors for local recurrence of resected colorectal lung metastases. Ann Thorac Surg. 2005;80(3):1040-5.
29. Saito Y, Omiya H, Kohno K, et al. Pulmonary metastasectomy for 165 patients with colorectal carcinoma: a prognostic assessment. J Thorac Cardiovasc Surg. 2002;124(5):1007-13.
30. Adam R, de Haas RJ, Wicherts DA, et al. Concomitant extrahepatic disease in patients with colorectal liver metastases: when is there a place for surgery? Ann Surg. 2011;253(2):349-59.
31. Huppertz A, Balzer T, Blakeborough A, et al. Improved detection of focal liver lesions at MR imaging: multicenter comparison of gadoxetic acid-enhanced MR images with intraoperative findings. Radiology. 2004;230(1):266-75.
32. Xu LH, Cai SJ, Cai GX, et al. Imaging diagnosis of colorectal liver metastases. World J Gastroenterol. 2011;17(42):4654-9.
33. Lesurtel M, Selzner M, Petrowsky H, et al. How should transection of the liver be performed? a prospective randomized study in 100 consecutive patients: comparing four different transection strategies. Ann Surg. 2005;242(6):814-22, discussion 822-3.
34. Simillis C, Constantinides VA, Tekkis PP, et al. Laparoscopic versus open hepatic resections for benign and malignant neoplasms—a meta-analysis. Surgery. 2007;141(2):203-11.
35. Wong SL, Mangu PB, Choti MA, et al. American Society of Clinical Oncology 2009 clinical evidence review on radiofrequency ablation of hepatic metastases from colorectal cancer. J Clin Oncol. 2010;28(3):493-508.
36. Ruers T, Punt C, Van Coevorden F, et al. Radiofrequency ablation combined with systemic treatment versus systemic treatment alone in patients with non-resectable colorectal liver metastases: a randomized EORTC Intergroup phase II study (EORTC 40004). Ann Oncol. 2012, Mar 19.
37. Mulier S, Ni Y, Jamart J, et al. Local recurrence after hepatic radiofrequency coagulation: multivariate meta-analysis and review of contributing factors. Ann Surg. 2005;242(2):158-71.
38. Pathak S, Jones R, Tang JM, et al. Ablative therapies for colorectal liver metastases: a systematic review. Colorectal Dis. 2011;13(9):e252-65.
39. Poston G, Adam R, Vauthey JN. Downstaging or downsizing: time for a new staging system in advanced colorectal cancer? J Clin Oncol. 2006;24(18):2702-6.
40. Folprecht G, Grothey A, Alberts S, et al. Neoadjuvant treatment of unresectable colorectal liver metastases: correlation between tumour response and resection rates. Ann Oncol. 2005;16(8):1311-9.
41. Adam R, Delvart V, Pascal G, et al. Rescue surgery for unresectable colorectal liver metastases downstaged by chemotherapy: a model to predict long-term survival. Ann Surg. 2004;240(4):644-57; discussion 657-8.

42. Folprecht G, Gruenberger T, Bechstein WO, et al. Tumour response and secondary resectability of colorectal liver metastases following neoadjuvant chemotherapy with cetuximab: the CELIM randomised phase 2 trial. Lancet Oncol. 2010;11(1):38-47.

43. Nordlinger B, Sorbye H, Glimelius B, et al. Perioperative chemotherapy with FOLFOX4 and surgery versus surgery alone for resectable liver metastases from colorectal cancer (EORTC Intergroup trial 40983): a randomised controlled trial. Lancet. 2008;371(9617):1007-16.

44. Adam R, Frilling A, Elias D, et al. Liver resection of colorectal metastases in elderly patients. Br J Surg. 2010;97(3):366-76.

45. Mitry E, Fields AL, Bleiberg H, et al. Adjuvant chemotherapy after potentially curative resection of metastases from colorectal cancer: a pooled analysis of two randomized trials. J Clin Oncol. 2008;26(30):4906-11.

46. Nordlinger B, Van Cutsem E, Gruenberger T, et al. Combination of surgery and chemotherapy and the role of targeted agents in the treatment of patients with colorectal liver metastases: recommendations from an expert panel. Ann Oncol. 2009;20(6):985-92.

47. Vauthey JN, Pawlik TM, Ribero D, et al. Chemotherapy regimen predicts steatohepatitis and an increase in 90-day mortality after surgery for hepatic colorectal metastases. J Clin Oncol. 2006;24(13):2065-72.

48. Rubbia-Brandt L, Audard V, Sartoretti P, et al. Severe hepatic sinusoidal obstruction associated with oxaliplatin-based chemotherapy in patients with metastatic colorectal cancer. Ann Oncol. 2004;15(3):460-6.

49. Karoui M, Penna C, Amin-Hashem M, et al. Influence of preoperative chemotherapy on the risk of major hepatectomy for colorectal liver metastases. Ann Surg. 2006;243(1):1-7.

50. Welsh FK, Tilney HS, Tekkis PP, et al. Safe liver resection following chemotherapy for colorectal metastases is a matter of timing. Br J Cancer. 2007;96(7):1037-42.

51. Mocellin S, Pilati P, Lise M, et al. Meta-analysis of hepatic arterial infusion for unresectable liver metastases from colorectal cancer: the end of an era? J Clin Oncol. 2007;25(35):5649-54.

52. Allen PJ, Nissan A, Picon AI, et al. Technical complications and durability of hepatic artery infusion pumps for unresectable colorectal liver metastases: an institutional experience of 544 consecutive cases. J Am Coll Surg. 2005;201(1):57-65.

53. Shitara K, Munakata M, Kudo T, et al. [Combination chemotherapy with hepatic arterial infusion of 5-fluorouracil (5-FU) and systemic irinotecan (CPT-11) in patients with unresectable liver metastases from colorectal cancer]. Gan To Kagaku Ryoho. 2006;33(13):2033-7.

54. Gallagher DJ, Capanu M, Raggio G, et al. Hepatic arterial infusion plus systemic irinotecan in patients with unresectable hepatic metastases from colorectal cancer previously treated with systemic oxaliplatin: a retrospective analysis. Ann Oncol. 2007;18(12):1995-9.

55. House MG, Kemeny NE, Gönen M, et al. Comparison of adjuvant systemic chemotherapy with or without hepatic arterial infusional chemotherapy after hepatic resection for metastatic colorectal cancer. Ann Surg. 2011;254(6):851-6.

56. Martin RC, Joshi J, Robbins K, et al. Hepatic intra-arterial injection of drug-eluting bead, irinotecan (DEBIRI) in unresectable colorectal liver metastases refractory to systemic chemotherapy: results of multi-institutional study. Ann Surg Oncol. 2011;18(1):192-8.

9 | Ischaemic Bowel

Keith Gardiner, William Wallace, Kevin McElvanna

DEFINITION

Intestinal ischaemia occurs when mesenteric perfusion is inadequate to meet intestinal metabolic demands for oxygen. Ischaemia may affect small or large bowel, or both, and may develop suddenly (acute mesenteric ischaemia) or gradually over months (chronic mesenteric ischaemia). Presentations vary from transient left-sided ischaemic colitis to devastating acute superior mesenteric arterial occlusion and full-thickness infarction of all small bowel and right colon.

MESENTERIC VASCULATURE

The gastrointestinal tract is supplied by three arteries. Coeliac axis supplies stomach, duodenum, liver, spleen and pancreas; superior mesenteric artery (SMA) supplies the duodenum, pancreas, small bowel and proximal colon (upto splenic flexure); inferior mesenteric artery (IMA) supplies the left colon and rectum. There are extensive collaterals and a high flow rate (approximately 20% of cardiac output). Venous drainage is via the inferior mesenteric vein (splenic vein) and superior mesenteric vein to the portal vein.

Splanchnic blood flow responds to vasodilators (nitric oxide, prostaglandins) and vasoconstrictors (catecholamines). Splanchnic vasoconstriction may be precipitated by hypovolaemic, haemorrhagic or septic shock, cardiac failure or by drugs.

AETIOLOGY OF INTESTINAL ISCHAEMIA

Aetiology may be classified as inadequate inflow (interrupted or inadequate supply), increased wall tension (high capillary pressure) or reduced venous outflow (Table 9.1).

TABLE 9.1: Classification of causes of intestinal ischaemia

Inadequate inflow		Increased wall tension	Reduced venous outflow
Interrupted/Occluded	*Non-occlusive*		
Embolism	Cardiogenic shock	Closed loop obstruction	Mesenteric vein thrombosis
Thrombosis	Hypovolaemia	Pseudo-obstruction	Mesenteric nodal disease
Volvulus	Sepsis		Pancreatic neoplasms
Mesenteric tears	Pancreatitis		
Abdominal aortic aneurysm surgery	Intra-abdominal hypertension		
Aortic dissection	Vasospasm due to drugs		
Strangulated hernia			

This chapter focuses on acute and chronic superior mesenteric ischaemia, due to occlusion of arterial inflow or venous outflow, and ischaemia resulting from low-flow states.

ACUTE SUPERIOR MESENTERIC ISCHAEMIA

Epidemiology

Acute superior mesenteric ischaemia (ASMI) is uncommon, accounting for 1–2 episodes/1,000 hospital admissions or 1–2% of gastrointestinal admissions. Mesenteric occlusion (embolus:thrombus 1.4:1) is the most common cause (68%) followed by non-occlusive mesenteric ischaemia (16%) and mesenteric vein thrombosis (16%).[1] Incidence increases with age and affects men and women equally.

Pathogenesis and Associations (Table 9.2)

Superior Mesenteric Artery Embolism

Emboli usually lodge at points of anatomical narrowing and are frequently found 3–10 cm distal to SMA origin (often beyond middle colic artery origin). Superior mesenteric artery embolism (SMAE) is associated with acute myocardial infarction, atrial fibrillation, cardiac thrombi (48%) and synchronous emboli (68%).[1]

Superior Mesenteric Artery Thrombosis

Thrombosis occurs in areas of atherosclerosis, near SMA origin or its main branches. Mesenteric atherosclerosis increases in frequency with age; prevalence is 20% in 65 year olds in Europe and North America.[2] Most patients with one stenotic mesenteric artery are asymptomatic.[3] Thrombotic occlusions are usually located more proximally than emboli, and as a result intestinal infarction is often more extensive.[1] Superior mesenteric artery thrombosis (SMAT) is usually a manifestation of generalised atherosclerosis (aortic, chronic mesenteric ischaemia, coronary artery, cerebrovascular and peripheral vascular disease),[4] and is also associated with disseminated cancer.

Non-Occlusive Mesenteric Ischaemia

Ischaemia occurs despite patent mesenteric arteries due to mesenteric vasospasm (vasopressin-angiotensin) and low blood flow. Mesenteric arterial stenosis is found in upto 40% of patients. Non-occlusive mesenteric ischaemia (NOMI) is seen in elderly, critically ill patients with severe cardiac disease, after cardiac surgery, or in patients who are septic and receiving high doses of inotropes. Other drugs have been implicated (digoxin, amphetamines, cocaine).[5] Synchronous infarction in liver, spleen and kidney is seen in 20% of patients.[1]

Superior Mesenteric Vein Thrombosis

Superior mesenteric vein thrombosis (SMVT) is associated with hyper-coaguable states (thrombophilia, oral contraceptive pill), previous thromboembolism, dehydration, obesity, inflammatory bowel disease, liver cirrhosis and intra-abdominal malignancy. It can develop postoperatively.[6]

TABLE 9.2: Associations with acute superior mesenteric ischaemia (ASMI)

Superior mesenteric artery embolism (SMAE)	Superior mesenteric artery thrombosis (SMAT)	Non-occlusive mesenteric ischaemia (NOMI)	Superior mesenteric vein thrombosis (SMVT)
Myocardial infarction	Aortic disease	Critically ill	Thrombophilia
Cardiac thrombosis	Coronary artery disease	Cardiac failure	Oral contraceptive pills
Atrial fibrillation	Cerebral infarction	Post-cardiac surgery	Thromboembolism
Synchronous emboli	Peripheral vascular disease	Sepsis	Dehydration
	Chronic mesenteric ischaemia	Inotropes	Obesity
	Disseminated cancer	Synchronous infarction of other organs	Inflammatory bowel disease
			Liver cirrhosis
			Intra-abdominal malignancy
			Postoperative

Clinical Presentation

Superior mesenteric artery occlusion (SMAE/SMAT) typically presents with sudden onset, severe abdominal pain, becoming progressively worse and associated with vomiting (70%) and diarrhoea (40–50%). The elderly may present with confusion and tachypnoea.

There may be no abdominal signs; the pain seeming out of keeping with physical findings. By the time bowel sounds disappear, the abdomen distends and there is guarding or rigidity, ischaemia will usually have progressed to transmural infarction. Superior mesenteric vein thrombosis and NOMI may present with vague abdominal pain, abdominal distension and diarrhoea.

Differential Diagnosis

The differential diagnosis is intestinal obstruction, perforated viscus, pancreatitis, cholecystitis, appendicitis and diverticulitis.

Diagnosis is often delayed due to non-specific presentation, and extensive infarction may develop. Therefore, this diagnosis should be considered and investigated in any patient with acute, severe, persistent (> 2 hours) and un-explained abdominal pain.

> **Key Point**
>
> Severe abdominal pain lasting longer than 2 hours, out of keeping with physical signs and without obvious cause should be investigated urgently for ASMI.

Investigations

Blood Tests

White blood cell count is usually raised ($10–14 \times 10^3$ cells/μL in 25% patients; 15–30 in 50% and > 30 in 25%). Other findings are metabolic acidosis, and elevations in phosphate (upto 80%), amylase (50%) and lactate. Elevated lactate is 100% sensitive, but only 42% specific for intestinal ischaemia/infarction. Elevated alpha glutathione s-transferase has 72% sensitivity and 77% specificity.[7]

Plain Radiology

Plain radiographs are most useful to exclude other causes of abdominal pain (obstruction, perforation) as findings in mesenteric ischaemia are non-specific (bowel distension or wall thickening). In advanced ischaemia, there may be air in the bowel wall (pneumatosis intestinalis) or portal vein (pneumatosis portalis).

Duplex Scanning of Mesenteric Vessels

Duplex imaging has a low sensitivity in acute ischaemia due to overlying bowel gas and low blood flow in acutely ill patients; thus is not recommended. Duplex scanning only assesses proximal SMA but emboli tend to lodge more distally.

Computed Tomography Angiography

Computed tomography (CT) angiography using multislice scanners can demonstrate mesenteric arterial stenoses or

occlusion, venous thrombosis, bowel wall thickening, mucosal enhancement, pneumatosis (intestinalis or portalis) and infarction of other organs, and can exclude other causes of abdominal pain (Figs 9.1 and 9.2). High positive and negative predictive values of 100% and 96% are reported.[8]

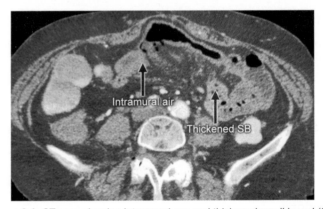

Figure 9.1: CT scan showing intramural gas and thickened small bowel (SB)

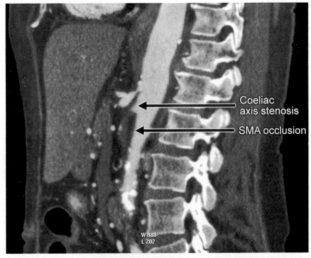

Figure 9.2: CT scan demonstrating coeliac axis stenosis and superior mesenteric artery (SMA) occlusion

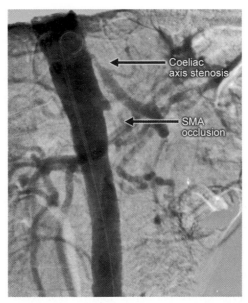

Figure 9.3: Mesenteric angiogram demonstrating coeliac stenosis and superior mesenteric artery (SMA) occlusion

Mesenteric Angiography

Angiography offers a sensitivity of 90–100% and a range of therapeutic options (intra-arterial vasodilators, thrombolysis, angioplasty and stenting). Disadvantages are invasiveness, limited emergency availability, contrast-associated nephrotoxicity and inability to assess intestinal infarction (Fig. 9.3).

Magnetic Resonance Angiography

Magnetic resonance angiography (MRA) is non-invasive (avoiding risks of contrast-associated allergic reactions and nephrotoxicity), mainly evaluates proximal coeliac and SMA (missing distal emboli), and may not identify low-flow states or secondary signs of acute ischaemia (bowel wall thickening).[9]

Diagnostic Laparoscopy

Diagnostic laparoscopy is less invasive than laparotomy. However, laparoscopy is unable to assess mucosal ischaemia, may have difficulty in assessing areas of doubtful bowel viability and may miss segmental ischaemia when 'running' the entire length of the bowel.[10]

CT angiography is the usual first investigation.

Treatment: General Measures

Oxygen, pain relief and broad-spectrum antibiotics are administered, haemodynamic and fluid/electrolyte/acid-base disturbances are corrected and

associated conditions are treated
(cardiac failure or arrhythmia).
Heparin is administered early
unless there is active bleeding.

> **Key Point**
>
> Urgent surgery is indicated for peritonitis irrespective of cause of acute mesenteric ischaemia.

Invasive monitoring in critical care is advised (hourly urine volume, central venous and arterial pressure). Patients need inotropes if fluid resuscitation fails to correct haemodynamic disturbances, although vasopressors may exacerbate mesenteric ischaemia.

Treatment: Specific Measures

Treatment depends on clinical findings and underlying cause. Peritonitis requires urgent laparotomy, but in its absence medical and endovascular options can be considered (Fig. 9.4).

Medical and Endovascular Treatments

Medical and endovascular approach depends on underlying aetiology:

Superior mesenteric artery occlusion (SMAE and SMAT): Endovascular management alone does not allow assessment for intestinal necrosis and should not be used if there is haemodynamic instability or peritonitis.

Arterial access is gained by femoral or brachial puncture; an aortogram defines anatomy and mesenteric arteries are selectively cannulated. Options

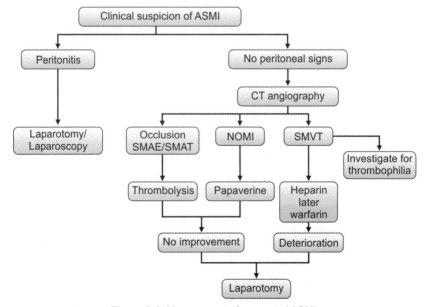

Figure 9.4: Management of suspected ASMI

Abbreviations: ASMI: Acute superior mesenteric ischaemia; SMAE: Superior mesenteric artery embolism; SMAT: Superior mesenteric artery thrombosis; NOMI: Non-occlusive mesenteric ischaemia; SMVT: Superior mesenteric vein thrombosis

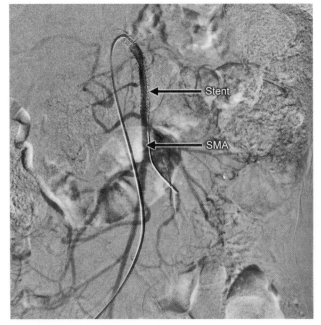

Figure 9.5: Superior mesenteric artery (SMA) revascularisation by stent

include aspiration embolectomy (for proximal SMAE), catheter-directed thrombolysis (use of tissue plasminogen activator to remove residual clot after embolectomy), mechanical thrombus fragmentation or stent insertion.

Angioplasty and stent insertion involves dilating a stenosis with an angioplasty balloon and insertion of a balloon-expandable stent (Fig. 9.5). Repeat angiography and pressure gradient measurement confirm a satisfactory result. After endovascular procedures, patients require critical care monitoring and serial abdominal examinations.

Non-occlusive mesenteric ischaemia: Treatment for NOMI is resuscitation, improvement of cardiac output and administration of intra-arterial vasodilators at the time of angiography (60 mg papaverine bolus followed by infusion 30–60 mg/h). Angiography is repeated after 24 hours to document improvement in vasospasm.[5] Papaverine can be continued for upto 5 days if vasospasm persists.

Superior mesenteric vein thrombosis: Aims of treatment are to stop extension of thrombosis and facilitate fibrinolysis. Rapid anticoagulation with heparin is necessary but risks intestinal bleeding when necrotic mucosa sloughs. Anticoagulation is successful in upto 90% of cases, although 32% patients may require small bowel resection.[11,12]

Patients require investigation for underlying causes (hypercoaguable state, liver cirrhosis). Warfarin is recommended for 3–6 months but is necessary lifelong for associated thrombophilia.[5] Surgery may be necessary subsequently

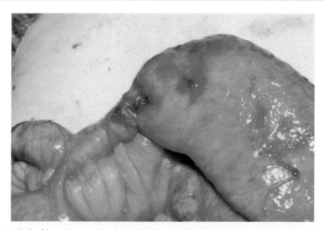

Figure 9.6: Chronic proximal small obstruction due to post-ischaemic stricture

due to stricture formation (Figure 9.6). Longer term, splanchnic vein recanalisation is reported in 45–92% of patients.[13] For all endovascular procedures, failure to improve or development of peritonitis mandates laparotomy.

> **Key Point**
>
> The aims of surgery for ASMI are to remove infarcted bowel, restore mesenteric blood flow and preserve as much small bowel as possible. Laparotomy for ASMI should involve both gastrointestinal and vascular surgeons.

Surgery

Urgent surgery is indicated for peritonitis irrespective of cause. The aims of surgery are to remove infarcted bowel, restore mesenteric flow and preserve small bowel. Laparotomy should be a joint procedure with gastrointestinal and vascular surgeons both present.

Abdomen, groins and thighs are prepared (potential for saphenous or femoral vein harvest). Through a midline incision, the abdomen should be thoroughly explored. Bowel is assessed by colour, sheen, peristalsis, visible and palpable mesenteric pulsations and bleeding from cut surfaces. Frankly necrotic bowel is obvious (Figs 9.7 and 9.8). Clinical criteria have a sensitivity of 82% and specificity of 91%.[14] Adjuncts that can be used are a Doppler ultrasound probe to assess mesenteric pulsatility, or fluorescein and a perfusion fluorometer.[14]

For patients with extensive intestinal necrosis, age, pre-existing functional state, co-morbidity, intraoperative stability and length of bowel that would remain are all considerations when deciding whether a procedure is futile. A second opinion is often valuable. Approximately, 50 cm of viable small bowel is required to sustain life if the colon is present. If the colon but less than 50 cm of small bowel is preserved, or less than 100 cm of small bowel remains in the absence of a colon, patients require life-long parenteral nutrition or need intestinal transplantation.

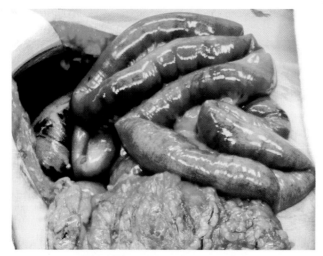

Figure 9.7: Diffuse ischaemia of small bowel and right colon due to superior mesenteric artery thrombosis (SMAT)

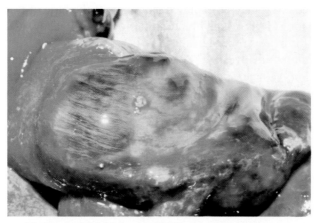

Figure 9.8: Patchy full-thickness small intestinal infarction in septic patient

Revascularisation should be considered first if there is no necrotic or perforated bowel as severely ischaemic intestine may become viable after revascularisation. Only frankly necrotic or perforated bowel should be removed initially.

Key Point

At laparotomy for ASMI, only bowel that is necrotic or perforated should be removed initially and intestine of dubious viability should be reassessed after revascularisation has been performed.

Intraoperative assessment of cause for ischaemia depends on distribution and extent of ischaemia and evaluation of SMA (palpation, handheld Doppler, intraoperative angiography) (Table 9.3).

TABLE 9.3: Appearances and superior mesenteric artery (SMA) pulse in acute superior mesenteric ischaemia (ASMI)

	Superior mesenteric artery thrombosis (SMAT)	Superior mesenteric artery embolism (SMAE)	Non-occlusive mesenteric ischaemia (NOMI)	Superior mesenteric vein thrombosis (SMVT)
Appearance	Pale contracted bowel		Patchy ischaemia	Congested, dilated bowel
Distribution	Affects all small bowel	Spares proximal bowel	Patchy throughout length	Diffuse or segmental
SMA pulse	Absent proximal pulse	Strong proximal but absent distal	Weak pulse along length	Good pulse along length

Intestinal revascularisation options are embolectomy, SMA bypass or retrograde SMA stenting. Superior mesenteric artery bypass is usually preferred for thrombosis as adequate thrombectomy in splanchnic arteries is difficult. The SMA may be explored anteriorly at the base of the transverse mesocolon for SMAE (usually more distal) or laterally above fourth part of duodenum for bypass procedures.

Embolectomy involves SMA control, longitudinal arteriotomy, systemic heparinisation, catheter embolectomy (3-4 Fr balloon catheter proximally; 2-3 Fr catheter distally in narrower vessels) and arteriotomy closure (suture or vein patch).

Emergency mesenteric bypass is usually by a single bypass (antegrade or retrograde) to the SMA. Choices for inflow are supracoeliac or infrarenal aorta, or common iliac artery. Retrograde bypass from infrarenal aorta or iliac artery is preferred due to easier exposure and avoidance of supramesenteric clamping and exacerbation of ischaemia. Choice of graft material [Dacron, externally supported polytetrafluoroethylene (PTFE), vein] depends on the presence of peritonitis and availability of vein. A reversed vein graft from long saphenous or femoral vein is preferred in the presence of peritonitis. Synthetic materials are easier to handle, less likely to kink and give a better size match.[15] Patency rates (at 3 years) depend on graft type (antegrade 93%; retrograde 95%; saphenous vein 95%; synthetic 89%).[16]

Retrograde open mesenteric stenting involves SMA exposure and control, longitudinal arteriotomy, thromboendarterectomy, retrograde insertion of a balloon expandable, covered stent and patch angioplasty with vein or bovine pericardium.[17] This hybrid technique combines laparotomy and bowel assessment with rapid revascularisation.[18]

Superior mesenteric vein thrombectomy has been infrequently described.

Intestinal viability is reassessed (inspection, pulses, Doppler) after revascularisation, but this is difficult due to low flow (hypovolaemia; hypotension), mesenteric vasospasm and reperfusion delay. Decisions about further resection should be delayed for 30 minutes to allow reperfusion.[19] Papaverine may be administered selectively to SMA to reduce vasospasm.

As much small bowel as possible is preserved (reducing risk of short bowel syndrome). Therefore, if in doubt, resection is deferred and a second-look laparotomy is performed 24 hours later. Transected bowel ends can be exteriorised or stapled closed and left within abdomen. Bowel resection rate is higher (53%) at second-look laparotomy compared to initial laparotomy and revascularisation (31%).[20]

Anastomosis after resection is safe if proximal and distal margins have good blood supply and the patient is haemodynamically stable. Anastomosis should not be performed (exteriorise or staple closed) if there is peritonitis or if revascularisation has been carried out.

Postoperatively, patients are transferred to critical care for monitoring and support to prevent secondary ischaemic events. Intestinal ischaemia-reperfusion results in a systemic inflammatory response and carries significant risk of multiorgan dysfunction.

Decisions regarding second-look laparotomy (or laparoscopy) are made during initial surgery. Indications include low flow state, intestinal anastomosis and mesenteric bypass.[21] At second-look laparotomy, it is usually clear what bowel needs resection.

> **Key Point**
>
> Second-look surgery should be planned during the first operation when there is low flow, intestine of dubious viability or if mesenteric bypass or intestinal anastomosis has been performed.

Outcome

Acute superior mesenteric ischaemia has a high perioperative mortality rate (32–69%) and low 5-year survival (18–50%).[15]

Mortality depends on cause, with in-hospital mortality being highest for NOMI, lower for acute SMA occlusion and lowest (20%) for SMVT.[1] Mortality is higher for SMAT than SMAE, possibly related to more proximal SMA occlusion with SMAT (more extensive bowel infarction).[22] The very high mortality found with NOMI (70%) is due to difficulties in diagnosis and in restoring haemodynamic stability.

Prompt diagnosis correlates with better survival.[23] Survival in patients with SMAE was 50% with early diagnosis (within 24 hours) but dropped to 30% with delay.[24] Surgical admission correlates with decreased mortality. Peritonitis and bowel necrosis at presentation are independent risk factors for death and parenteral nutrition dependency. Short bowel syndrome may result in upto 23% of patients.[25]

> **Key Point**
>
> Acute superior mesenteric ischaemia has a high mortality rate. Survival is related to underlying cause, and speed of diagnosis and intervention.

A lower mortality rate (15.6%) is described with angioplasty +/- stent compared with surgical bypass (27.6%) in a non-randomised study.[26]

CHRONIC SUPERIOR MESENTERIC ISCHAEMIA

Epidemiology

Chronic superior mesenteric ischaemia (CSMI) is a relatively rare cause of hospital admission (1/100,000; 1–2% of gastrointestinal admissions).[27]

Pathogenesis and Associations

Atherosclerosis causing SMA stenosis or occlusion is the most common cause. It is associated with smoking, diabetes, hyperlipidaemia, peripheral vascular disease (72%), hypertension (66%) and coronary artery disease (58%). Mesenteric atherosclerosis usually extends from the aortic wall and is therefore found near vessel origin. Atherosclerosis most commonly affects the coeliac artery (90%) followed by IMA (56%) and SMA (43%); 21% of patients have stenosis of all three vessels.[28]

Patients with CSMI mostly have critical SMA stenosis (>70%) in addition to stenosis of at least one other vessel, disrupting collateral blood supply. Other causes of chronic mesenteric ischaemia are fibrodysplasia, vasculitis, Takayasu's disease and SMVT.

Acute ischaemia can complicate CSMI and carries a higher mortality. Symptoms of CSMI are present in 43% of patients with acute SMA occlusion[29] and one-third of patients with multivessel stenoses progress to intestinal infarction.[30]

> **Key Point**
>
> Chronic superior mesenteric ischaemia needs to be investigated and treated to prevent the high morbidity and mortality associated with acute thrombosis.

Clinical Presentation

Patients usually present in their 60s and 70s with a colicky, post-prandial epigastric pain (mesenteric angina) and un-intentional weight loss (10–15 kg by diagnosis).

> **Key Point**
>
> Chronic superior mesenteric ischaemia is characterised by colicky post-prandial abdominal pain and progressive weight loss.

Examination may reveal cachexia, smoking-related chest disease, scaphoid abdomen scarred by erythema ab igne, abdominal bruit or reduced/absent peripheral pulses.

Differential diagnoses include biliary disease and peptic ulcer.

Investigations

Duplex Ultrasonography

Duplex ultrasonography is non-invasive and not contraindicated with renal disease (avoids intravenous contrast), but obesity and bowel gas can inhibit its accuracy. Criteria for CSMI are peak systolic flow, end-diastolic velocity and retrograde flow in hepatic artery (coeliac stenosis).

Mesenteric Angiography

Mesenteric angiography is the femoral or brachial approach to demonstrate arterial stenoses or anatomical variations, distal flow and collateralisation. Its major advantage is therapeutic potential (stent insertion). Disadvantages include arterial dissection, bleeding or contrast-related nephropathy. Contrast angiography is used to assess significant disease identified on Duplex or in patients too obese to permit reliable Duplex assessment.

Computed Tomography Angiography

Computed tomography angiography is the non-invasive demonstration of arterial stenoses, organ perfusion, aortic pathology, iliac tortuosity and other diseases without risk of arterial trauma or dissection. It has a high sensitivity and specificity (95%) for identifying mesenteric arterial stenoses[31] but carries the risk of contrast-induced nephropathy and does not permit interventions.

Magnetic Resonance Angiography

Magnetic resonance angiography with gadolinium enhancement has a high sensitivity and specificity (95%)[32] but concerns exist over gadolinium-associated systemic fibrosis and renal failure.[31]

Patients with CSMI should undergo upper and lower gastrointestinal endoscopy (if not already carried out). Specific first-line investigation is usually Duplex ultrasonography or CT angiography followed by mesenteric angiography.

Diagnosis

Chronic superior mesenteric ischaemia is diagnosed by typical symptoms, and duplex ultrasonographic evidence of occlusion or high-grade stenoses of SMA and coeliac artery (peak systolic velocity of > 275 and 200 cm/s respectively).[33]

Treatment

Aims of treatment are to relieve symptoms, restore weight and prevent intestinal infarction. Mesenteric revascularisation is indicated for symptomatic disease.[34]

The decision to treat CSMI depends on symptom severity, presence of multivessel disease and severity of stenoses.[31]

Options are endovascular mesenteric angioplasty and stenting or open revascularisation. Transaortic endarterectomy is rarely used.[33]

Mesenteric angioplasty (via femoral or brachial approaches), with angioplasty alone for short, non-ostial, focal stenoses; angioplasty and a balloon expandable stent are deployed for long occlusions flush with the aorta. Stenting has a higher technical success than angioplasty, but symptomatic relief, restenosis rates, morbidity and mortality are similar.[35]

Where two or more vessels are critically stenosed, SMA revascularisation is usually of greatest benefit. If SMA revascularisation is not technically possible, angioplasty or stenting of the coeliac axis or IMA may benefit.[36,37]

Open mesenteric bypass may be antegrade or retrograde, single or multiple vessel, with an aortic- or iliac-based origin.[33] Supracoeliac, bifurcated, polyester graft from the aorta to the coeliac axis and SMA was the choice in of 80% open mesenteric reconstructions.[29,38] The iliac artery is a better choice in the elderly due to calcified or diseased aortas. Retrograde SMA stents avoid the need for extensive dissection, vein harvesting and the use of prosthetic grafts in those with extensive aortoiliac disease.[18]

Endovascular stents are used in 70% of patients with CSMI,[33] open bypass being reserved for failed percutaneous intervention, occluded or stenosed stents.

Non-atherosclerotic mesenteric arterial disease (e.g. vasculitis) usually requires surgical bypass as lesions are long and do not respond well to angioplasty.[33]

> **Key Point**
>
> In CSMI, mesenteric angioplasty and stenting have a high success (90–95%) and a lower peri-procedure mortality and morbidity than open mesenteric bypass. Open mesenteric bypass has a lower restenosis and symptomatic recurrence rate than mesenteric angioplasty and stenting.

Outcome

Both endovascular and open mesenteric bypass deliver excellent symptom relief (up to 97% of patients).[33]

1. Endovascular success is 90–95%.[35] Peri-procedure mortality rate is 3–5% and morbidity is 20%.[26,35] Risks of endovascular procedures include puncture site problems, contrast-induced nephrotoxicity, arterial dissection and distal embolisation. Arterial dissection or vessel rupture can be managed using covered stents, whilst distal embolisation may respond to thrombolysis or thromboaspiration. Both conditions can lead to acute mesenteric ischaemia, necessitating emergency laparotomy. Patency rates at 12 months are 65–85%, whilst restenosis has been reported to occur in almost one-third of patients,[26] and can lead to recurrent symptoms or acute mesenteric ischaemia.[35,39,40] Symptomatic restenoses are treated by repeat angioplasty or open bypass.

2. Open mesenteric bypass leads to less restenosis, symptomatic recurrences and re-interventions compared with mesenteric angioplasty and stent insertion. However, there is a higher mortality $(0-15\%)^{33}$ and morbidity (10–38%) due to cardiac and pulmonary complications $(10-38\%)$.[26,33]

Endovascular procedures are preferred in patients who have suitable lesions.[26,33]

CONCLUSIONS

Acute superior mesenteric ischaemia is often diagnosed late and has a high mortality. An improved outcome is seen with early diagnosis and intervention. Therefore, patients with severe abdominal pain, out of keeping with signs and with no other obvious cause require urgent investigation. The investigation of choice is CT angiography.

The priorities for management of ASMI are:

1. Recognition (high index of suspicion)
2. Resuscitation
3. Revascularisation
4. Resection of intestine (limited initially to necrotic and perforated bowel)
5. Reassessment (after revascularisation and at second-look laparotomy)
6. Reduction of recurrence (critical care postoperatively to prevent secondary ischaemia; long-term anticoagulation)

Key Points for Clinical Practice

1. Severe abdominal pain lasting longer than 2 hours, out of keeping with physical signs and without obvious cause should be investigated urgently for ASMI.

2. CT angiography is the investigation of choice for ASMI.

3. Urgent surgery is indicated for peritonitis irrespective of cause of acute mesenteric ischaemia.

4. The aims of surgery for ASMI are to remove infarcted bowel, restore mesenteric blood flow and preserve as much small bowel as possible. Laparotomy for ASMI should involve both gastrointestinal and vascular surgeons.

5. At laparotomy for ASMI, only bowel that is necrotic or perforated should be removed initially, and intestine of dubious viability should be reassessed after revascularisation has been performed.

6. Second-look surgery should be planned during the first operation when there is low flow, intestine of dubious viability, or if mesenteric bypass or intestinal anastomosis has been performed.

7. Acute superior mesenteric ischaemia has a high mortality. Survival is related to underlying cause, and speed of diagnosis and intervention.

8. Chronic superior mesenteric ischaemia needs to be investigated and treated to prevent the high morbidity and mortality associated with acute thrombosis.

9. Chronic superior mesenteric ischaemia is characterised by colicky post-prandial abdominal pain and progressive weight loss.

10. In CSMI, mesenteric angioplasty and stenting have a high success (90–95%) and a lower peri-procedure mortality and morbidity than open mesenteric bypass. Open mesenteric bypass has a lower restenosis and symptomatic recurrence rate than mesenteric angioplasty and stenting.

Chronic superior mesenteric ischaemia is often diagnosed late and can be complicated by ASMI. It should be investigated and treated urgently to reduce the high mortality associated with ASMI. Investigation of choice is Duplex ultrasound followed by mesenteric angiography. Chronic superior mesenteric ischaemia can be successfully treated by endovascular techniques and by open surgery. Endovascular techniques are preferred in patients who have suitable lesions due to lower morbidity and mortality.

REFERENCES

1. Acosta S. Epidemiology of mesenteric vascular disease: clinical implications. Semin Vasc Surg. 2010;23:4-8.
2. Roobottom CA, Dubbins PA. Significant disease of the celiac and superior mesenteric arteries in asymptomatic patients: predictive value of Doppler sonography. AJR Am J Roentgenol. 1993;161:985-8.
3. Brandt LJ, Boley SJ. AGA technical review on intestinal ischemia. American Gastrointestinal Association. Gastroenterology. 2000;118:954-68.
4. Acosta S, Sonesson B, Resch T. Endovascular therapeutic approaches for acute superior mesenteric artery occlusion. Cardiovasc Intervent Radiol. 2009;32:896-905.
5. Kozuch PL, Brandt LJ. Diagnosis and management of mesenteric ischaemia with an emphasis on pharmacotherapy. Aliment Pharmacol Ther. 2005;21:201-15.
6. Acosta S, Ogren M, Sternby NH, et al. Mesenteric venous thrombosis with transmural intestinal infarction: a population-based study. J Vasc Surg. 2005;41:59-63.
7. Acosta S, Nilsson T. Current status on plasma biomarkers for acute mesenteric ischaemia. J Thromb Thrombolysis. 2012;33:355-61.
8. Aschoff AJ, Stuber G, Becker BW, et al. Evaluation of acute mesenteric ischemia: accuracy of biphasic mesenteric multi-detector CT angiography. Abdom Imaging. 2009;34:345-57.
9. Laissy JP, Trillaud H, Douek P. MR angiography: Noninvasive vascular imaging of the abdomen. Abdom Imaging. 2002;27:488-506.
10. Sauerland S, Agresta F, Bergamaschi R, et al. Laparoscopy for abdominal emergencies: evidence-based guidelines of the European Association for Endoscopic Surgery. Surg Endosc. 2006;20:14-29.
11. Brunaud L, Antunes L, Collinet-Adler S, et al. Acute mesenteric venous thrombosis: case for nonoperative management. J Vasc Surg. 2001;34:673-9.
12. Morasch MD, Ebaugh JL, Chiou AC, et al. Mesenteric venous thrombosis: a changing clinical entity. J Vasc Surg. 2001;34:680-4.
13. Amitrano L, Guardascione MA, Scaglione M, et al. Prognostic factors in noncirrhotic patients with splanchnic vein thrombosis. Am J Gastroenterol. 2007;102:2464-70.
14. Bulkley GB, Zuidema GD, Hamilton SR, et al. Intraoperative determination of small intestinal viability following ischemic injury: a prospective, controlled trial of two adjuvant methods (Doppler and fluorescein) compared with standard clinical judgement. Ann Surg. 1981;193:628-37.
15. Wyers MC. Acute mesenteric ischaemia: diagnostic approach and surgical treatment. Semin Vasc Surg. 2010;23:9-20.
16. McMillan WD, McCarthy WJ, Bresticker MR, et al. Mesenteric artery bypass: objective patency determination. J Vasc Surg. 1995;21:729-41.

17. Wyers MC, Powell RJ, Nolan BW, et al. Retrograde mesenteric stenting during laparotomy for acute occlusive mesenteric ischemia. J Vasc Surg. 2007;45:269-75.

18. Kibbe MR, Hassoun HT. Acute mesentric ischaemia. Part 6 (Vascular System) Chapter 4 In ACS Surgery: Principles and Practice; S Ahsley (ed). 2010 Decker Publishing.

19. Kazmers A. Operative management of acute mesenteric ischemia. Ann Vasc Surg. 1998;12:187-97.

20. Kougias P, Lau D, El Sayed HF, et al. Determinants of mortality and treatment outcome following surgical interventions for acute mesenteric ischemia. J Vasc Surg. 2007;46:467-74.

21. Yanar H, Taviloglu K, Ertekin C, et al. Planned second-look laparotomy in the management of acute mesenteric ischemia. World J Gastroenterol. 2007;13:3350-3.

22. Hassoun HT, Fischer UM, Attuwaybi BO, et al. Regional hypothermia reduces mucosal NF-kappaB and PMN priming via gut lymph during canine mesenteric ischemia/reperfusion. J Surg Res. 2003;115:121-6.

23. Giulini S, Bonardelli S, Cangiotti L, et al. Factors affecting prognosis in acute intestinal ischemia. Int Angiol. 1987;6:415-20.

24. Boley SJ, Feinstein FR, Sammartano R, et al. New concepts in the management of emboli of the superior mesenteric artery. Surg Gynecol Obstet. 1981;153:561-9.

25. Rhee RY, Gloviczki P, Mendonca CT, et al. Mesenteric venous thrombosis: still a lethal disease in the 1990s. J Vasc Surg. 1994;20:688-97.

26. Schermerhorn ML, Giles KA, Hamdan AD, et al. Mesenteric revascularization: management and outcomes in the United States, 1988-2006. J Vasc Surg. 2009;50:341-8.

27. Mitchell EL, Moneta GL. Mesenteric duplex scanning. Perspect Vasc Surg Endovasc Ther. 2006;18:175-83.

28. Thomas JH, Blake K, Pierce GE, et al. The clinical course of asymptomatic mesenteric arterial stenosis. J Vasc Surg. 1998;27:840-4.

29. Park WM, Cherry KJ Jr, Chua HK, et al. Current results of open revascularization for chronic mesenteric ischemia: a standard for comparison. J Vasc Surg. 2002;35:853-9.

30. Kolkman JJ, Mensink PB, van Petersen AS, et al. Clinical approach to chronic gastrointestinal ischaemia: from 'intestinal angina' to the spectrum of chronic splanchnic disease. Scand J Gastroenterol Suppl. 2004;241:9-16.

31. Chandra A, Quinones-Baldrich WJ. Chronic mesenteric ischemia: how to select patients for invasive treatment. Semin Vasc Surg. 2010;23:21-8.

32. Meaney JF, Prince MR, Nostrant TT, et al. Gadolinium-enhanced MR angiography of visceral arteries in patients with suspected chronic mesenteric ischemia. J Magn Reson Imaging. 1997;1:171-6.

33. Oderich GS, Gloviczki P, Bower TC. Open surgical treatment for chronic mesenteric ischemia in the endovascular era: when is it necessary and what is the preferred technique? Semin Vasc Surg. 2010;23:36-46.

34. Wilson DB, Mostafavi K, Craven TE, et al. Clinical course of mesenteric artery stenosis in elderly Americans. Arch Intern Med. 2006;166:2095-100.

35. Kougias P, El Sayed HF, et al. Management of chronic mesenteric ischemia. The role of endovascular therapy. J Endovascular Therapy. 2007;14:395-405.

36. Alam A, Uberoi R. Chronic mesenteric ischemia treated by isolated angioplasty of the inferior mesenteric artery. Cardiovasc Intervent Radiol. 2005;28:536-8.

37. Landis MS, Rajan DK, Simons ME, et al. Percutaneous management of chronic mesenteric ischemia: outcomes after intervention. J Vasc Interv Radiol. 2005;16:1319-25.

38. Oderich GS, Bower TC, Sullivan TM, et al. Open versus endovascular revascularisation for chronic mesenteric ischemia: risk-stratified outcomes. J Vasc Surg. 2009;49:1472-9.

39. Atkins MD, Kwolek CJ, LaMuraglia GM, et al. Surgical revascularization versus endovascular therapy for chronic mesenteric ischemia: a comparative experience. J Vasc Surg. 2007;45:1162-71.

40. Davies RS, Wall ML, Silverman SH, et al. Surgical versus endovascular reconstruction for chronic mesenteric ischemia: a contemporary UK series. Vasc Endovascular Surg. 2009;43:157-64.

10 | Anal Cancer

Jurgen J Mulsow, P Ronan O'Connell

INTRODUCTION

The anal canal extends from the anorectal junction to the anal margin where the non-keratinised squamous epithelium meets the perianal hair-bearing skin. Cancer of the anal canal is rare in the general population, accounting for only 4% of large bowel malignancies. Its incidence is increased in individuals with known risk factors including a history of immunosuppression, human papilloma virus (HPV) infection, smoking, and in men who have sex with men (MSM). The majority (approximately 80%) of anal cancers arise from the squamous mucosa of the anal canal and perianal skin. Anal intraepithelial neoplasia (AIN) is a known precursor for the development of anal squamous cell carcinoma (SCC). In patients with established anal cancer, treatment is multidisciplinary and primarily nonoperative. In Europe, the overall 5-year survival for patients with SCC is 60%, and 46% for individuals with adenocarcinoma of the anus.[1]

EPIDEMIOLOGY

The age standardised incidence rate for anal cancer in Europe is 8.9 per million population.[1] Geographically, the prevalence of anal cancer varies widely, and is higher in those areas where cervical, penile and vulval tumours are relatively more common. The incidence of anal cancer is also increasing in line with the increasing incidence of human immunodeficiency virus (HIV) infection, particularly in younger age groups. Anal cancer is more common in females (male:female ratio 1:3)[1] and has a peak incidence at approximately 60 years of age.

RISK FACTORS

A number of predisposing risk factors for the development of anal cancer have been identified. The incidence is highest in MSM, particularly those who are HIV positive. Homosexual men are 20 times more likely to develop anal cancer than heterosexual men.

Human papilloma virus infection is found in the majority (> 70%) of individuals with invasive anal cancer.[2] The high incidence of anal cancer in geographical areas that also display high incidences of other HPV-associated cancers suggests a shared or common aetiology. The HPV types most commonly associated with anal cancer are HPV-16 and HPV-18. Most individuals with anal cancer who are positive for HPV are positive for HPV-16 (87%), whilst only 6% are positive for HPV-18.[2] The prevalence of HPV-16 and HPV-18 is significantly higher in HIV positive individuals than in those who are HIV negative—three quarters of HIV positive MSM are found to have high-risk HPV types.[3]

Genital warts were recently shown in a large Danish study to be an independent risk factor for the development of anal cancer. In men with genital warts, the standardised incidence ratio for the development of anal cancer was 21.5, whilst that in females was 7.8.[4] Genital warts are typically caused by non-oncogenic HPV types 6 and 11. It is hypothesised that individuals with genital warts are also likely to harbour oncogenic HPV types, hence the increased incidence of anogenital cancers.

Immunosuppression, particularly when associated with HIV infection, is associated with an increased risk for the development of anal cancer. HIV-infected MSM have an unadjusted anal cancer incidence rate of 131/100,000 person-years. For other HIV-infected men, the incidence rate is 46, whilst that in HIV-uninfected men is 2/100,000 person-years. In HIV-infected women, the anal cancer rate is 30/100,000 person-years.[5]

A recent Swedish study involving over 300,000 individuals followed for 37 years demonstrated an increased risk of anal cancer amongst smokers (hazard ratio 2.4).[6] Smokers also appear to be at increased risk of disease recurrence following treatment and carry an overall worse prognosis.[7,8]

Anal intraepithelial neoplasia is strongly associated with the presence of HPV infection (typically serotypes 6, 11, 16, 18) and may progress to invasive SCC. The disease process is analogous to the development of cervical cancer in individuals with cervical intraepithelial neoplasia (CIN), although the rate of malignant transformation appears lower. The incidence of AIN in the general population is less than 1% but is increased in immunocompromised individuals, women with a history of CIN and individuals with extensive genital warts.[9] A recent meta-analysis showed a pooled prevalence for high grade AIN of 29.1% in HIV-positive MSM, and 21.5% in HIV-negative MSM.[3]

Anal intraepithelial neoplasia I and II (low-grade dysplasia) are characterised by cellular atypia, which is confined to the lower two-thirds of the epithelium, whereas the changes in AIN III (high-grade dysplasia) are seen throughout the full thickness of the epithelium. Calculation of the rate of progression from high-grade AIN to invasive cancer is difficult due to the lack of large published series with extensive

Key Point

Anal cancer is more common in individuals with risk factors including a history of immunosuppression, HPV infection, smoking, anal dysplasia and in MSM.

follow-up. Machalek et al performed a meta-analysis of published data and calculated theoretical progression rates for high-grade AIN of approximately 1 in 600 per year in HIV-positive MSM, and 1 in 4,000 for HIV-negative MSM.[3] By comparison, the rate of progression to invasive cancer in women with CIN III is 1/80 per year.

SCREENING AND VACCINATION FOR ANAL CANCER

Presently, screening for anal cancer is confined to individuals at very high risk and is performed only in highly specialised centres. The reasons for this are threefold: first, the limited available data suggest that the progression rate to invasive disease for AIN is low; second, there are inadequate data to show that treatment of high-grade anal dysplasia will lead to a reduction in the incidence of anal cancer; third, an acceptable, reliable and widely available screening test is not yet available.

Vaccination may in future offer a means of reducing the rate of anal cancer in high-risk individuals. A recent randomised trial showed that vaccination with the quadrivalent HPV vaccine significantly reduces the incidence of AIN in MSM.[10] Whether this will translate to reduced incidences of anal cancer requires longer-term follow-up.

PATHOLOGY

The World Health Organization classification of anal cancer is outlined in Table 10.1. Squamous cell carcinoma and adenocarcinoma account for more than 95% of cases,[1] with the majority of tumours (approximately 80%) arising in the squamous mucosa of the anal canal and perianal skin (Fig. 10.1). Squamous cell carcinoma arising in the anal canal should be distinguished from that of the anal margin, the latter having a more indolent course. Squamous cell carcinoma was at one time sub-classified as either basaloid, keratinising or non-keratinising. Distinguishing these subtypes is challenging and all share a similar prognosis. Hence, current recommendations advise the use of the term 'squamous cell carcinoma'. Adenocarcinoma of the anus is a less common variant thought to arise in the anal glands. Most reports suggest that adenocarcinoma accounts for less than 10% of anal cancers; however, a recent Europe-based review reported an incidence rate of 25%.[1] This discrepancy may reflect the difficulty in discriminating true adenocarcinoma of the anus from a low rectal tumour invading the anal canal.

Precancerous lesions of the anus may be classified as squamous dysplasia of the anal canal (AIN I–III), squamous dysplasia of the anal margin (Bowen's disease) and Paget's

> **Key Point**
>
> Squamous cell carcinoma of the anal canal must be distinguished from that of the anal margin as the staging, treatment and prognosis differ according to the site.

TABLE 10.1: Classzification of tumours of the anal canal

1. Epithelial tumours
a. Intraepithelial neoplasia (dysplasia)
b. Carcinoma
Squamous cell carcinoma (SCC)
Adenocarcinoma
Mucinous carcinoma
Small cell carcinoma
Undifferentiated carcinoma
Others
c. Carcinoid tumour
2. Malignant melanoma
3. Non-epithelial tumours
4. Secondary tumours

Source: Adapted from Fenger et al. Tumours of the anal canal. In: World Health Organization Classification of Tumours Pathology and Genetics of the Digestive System. Lyon, France: IARC Press; 2000. pp. 145-56.

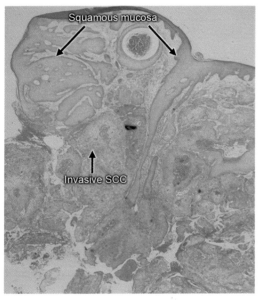

Figure 10.1: Invasive moderately differentiated squamous cell carcinoma (SCC) arising from anal squamous mucosa (2x) *Courtesy*: Ciara Barrett, Dublin

disease of the anus. Approximately, 50% of patients with Paget's disease have synchronous or metachronous internal tumours, whilst 50% develop invasive disease in the primary lesion.

Anal cancer spread is typically via the lymphatics. Distal anal tumours spread to the inguinal nodes, whilst more proximal tumours spread via the mesorectal nodes. Approximately, 10–15% of patients have inguinal metastases at presentation, the risk increasing with tumour T-stage.

CLINICAL FEATURES

Patients with anal cancer may have local symptoms including discomfort, pruritus, discharge or bleeding. A palpable lesion or mass may be evident, and in advanced cases faecal incontinence may be a feature. Examination typically reveals an ulcerating nodular lesion. Patients with AIN may have similar symptoms, and examination may be characterised by the presence of white plaque-like lesions that may be raised.

INVESTIGATION AND STAGING FOR SUSPECTED ANAL INTRAEPITHELIAL NEOPLASIA AND ANAL CANCER

Investigation begins with clinical examination and should distinguish tumours arising in the anal canal from those of the anal margin. Further staging through radiological imaging aims to detect local and distant disease and determine whether treatment may be undertaken with curative intent. Staging follows the guidelines of the American Joint Committee on Cancer (AJCC) 7th edition for anal canal (Table 10.2). The 6th edition guidelines still apply to the classification of anal margin tumours. For anal margin tumours, T4 designates invasion of the deep extradermal structures whilst involvement of regional nodes is designated N1.

TABLE 10.2: American Joint Committee on Cancer (AJCC) 7th edition staging of tumours of the anal canal

Primary tumour (T)	
TX	Tumour cannot be assessed
T0	No evidence of tumour
Tis	Carcinoma *in situ*, including AIN II-III
T1	Tumour < 2 cm in dimension
T2	Tumour 2–5 cm in dimension
T3	Tumour > 5 cm
T4	Tumour of any size, invading adjacent organs
Regional nodes	
NX	Nodes cannot be assessed
N0	No nodal metastases
N1	Perirectal node metastases
N2	Unilateral internal iliac and/or inguinal node metastases
N3	Perirectal and inguinal node metastases and/or bilateral internal iliac and/or inguinal node metastases
Metastases	
M0	No distant metastases
M1	Distant metastases

Anal Intraepithelial Neoplasia

A diagnosis of AIN requires biopsy and histopathological examination of suspicious lesions. At the time of assessment, multiple biopsies of the anal canal should be taken to determine the exact extent of the dysplasia, a process known as anal mapping. Cytological assessment is less reliable, particularly when diagnosing high-grade dysplasia.[11] Anal dysplasia may be detected *in vivo* using anoscopy combined with 3–5% aqueous acetic acid and Lugol's iodine.[9] This technique is highly specialised and is currently restricted to centres performing high volumes of investigation in individuals at increased risk.

Anal Cancer

Patients with suspected anal cancer should undergo formal examination under anaesthesia and biopsy of the suspicious lesion. The site of the lesion should be carefully noted, in particular, distinguishing tumours arising in the anal canal from those of the anal margin. The inguinal nodes should be palpated and fine needle aspiration cytology (FNAC) or biopsy should be performed in cases where these nodes are found to be enlarged. Clinical assessment of the inguinal nodes is however unreliable. Ultrasound of the groin in combination with FNAC of suspicious nodes may improve nodal staging accuracy but as yet data to support routine use are lacking. Whilst computed tomography (CT) of the thorax, abdomen and pelvis is routinely performed to detect intra-abdominal or distant metastases, there are few data to define the accuracy of CT in staging the inguinal nodes in patients with anal cancer.

Computed tomography when combined with [^{18}F] fluorodeoxyglucose positron emission tomography (PET) appears to have greater sensitivity for the detection of metastatic lymph nodes. PET/CT may alter the disease stage in 36–42% of patients when compared to conventional staging modalities.[12,13] There are limited available data to allow correlation between PET/CT and findings at histological examination. Such data as there are suggest a significant false positive rate with PET/CT for the detection of nodal disease (specificity 80%).[14] Despite this potential limitation, PET/CT is recommended routinely by the National Comprehensive Cancer Network treatment guidelines for the staging of anal cancer due to its sensitivity in detecting involved nodes.[15]

Whilst endoanal ultrasound may be of use in the staging of early anal tumours, it is limited in its ability to stage nodal disease.[16] Magnetic resonance imaging (MRI) allows reliable local tumour and nodal staging,[16] and should ideally be employed in combination with CT in the staging of all patients with anal cancer (Figs 10.2A and B).[17,18]

Sentinel node biopsy has been investigated as a means of improving nodal staging accuracy in patients with anal cancer. The technique is feasible with

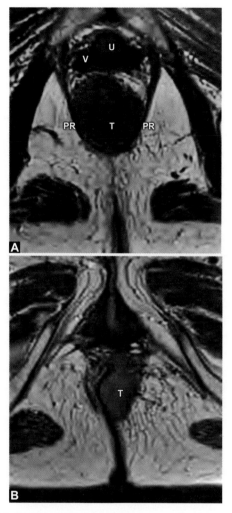

Figures 10.2A and B: (A) Axial T2-weighted magnetic resonance imaging demonstrating circumferential thickening of the anorectal junction at the level of the puborectalis muscle; (B) Axial T2-weighted image of the perineum demonstrating asymmetrical thickening of the anal margin at the level of the subcutaneous component of the external anal sphincter to the left of the midline consistent with tumour.
Abbreviations: U: Urethra; V: Vagina; PR: Puborectalis muscle; T: Tumour
Courtesy: Tony Geoghegan, Dublin

high sentinel node detection rates (upto 100%)[19] and has been shown to alter stage in upto 25% of patients.[14] As with PET/CT, the interpretation of results for sentinel node mapping in anal cancer must allow for the lack of

Key Point

Staging of the patient with anal cancer should include examination under anaesthesia, CT of thorax/abdomen/pelvis and MRI of pelvis. PET/CT is increasingly useful in the initial staging, particularly for the identification of nodal disease.

histopathological data to validate the accuracy of the technique in staging the nodal basin as a whole.

TREATMENT

Treatment of Anal Intraepithelial Neoplasia

Patients with low-grade dysplasia (AIN I or II) may be managed expectantly with observation alone due to the low rate of progression to invasive disease. It is suggested that long-term follow-up is unnecessary in this group.

Anal intraepithelial neoplasia III carries a higher risk of conversion to invasive cancer; however, the overall risk remains low. In this group, the treatment choice is primarily between observation and local excision. Local excision is particularly suited to focal (less than one-third of the circumference of the anus) symptomatic lesions.[9] Excision of wider areas is not advocated due to the risk of subsequent anal stenosis. Furthermore, complete excision of all dysplastic tissue is difficult to achieve (reported as occurring in less than 50% of cases) and rapid recurrence of high-grade dysplasia may be seen in 60% of patients.[20] Patients with HIV are at particularly high risk of recurrence following surgical eradication. Thus, patients with multifocal disease should undergo excision of the symptomatic area alone, and have 6-monthly assessment of any residual lesion.[9]

Imiquimod, a topically applied immunomodulator, has been shown to cause regression of high-grade dysplasia and it may be considered in the management of patients with multifocal AIN III.[9,21]

Ablative therapies including cryotherapy, laser and electro-cautery are associated with significant postoperative pain and high recurrence rates and are rarely used.

> **Key Point**
>
> Patients with focal high-grade dysplasia should undergo surgical excision; those with multifocal disease should undergo excision of symptomatic lesions alone.

Treatment of Squamous Cell Carcinoma of the Anal Margin

The treatment of early tumours (T1-2) is wide local excision. Additional radiation to the pelvis and inguinal nodes may be considered for more advanced cases and typically will be accompanied by systemic chemotherapy. A combination of surgical excision followed by definitive radiotherapy (either external beam or brachytherapy) is associated with a 5-year locoregional control rate of 78%, a sphincter preservation rate of 80% and overall survival of 55% at 5 years.[22] Abdominoperineal excision may be necessary for patients with tumour involvement of the anal sphincter and/or those who have not responded to initial therapy.

Buschke-Lowenstein disease, a rare well-differentiated SCC arising in perianal condylomata, may be treated by wide local excision.

Treatment of Squamous Cell Carcinoma of the Anal Canal

Chemoradiotherapy is now the standard approach to the management of SCC of the anus. The aims of treatment are local control whilst preserving sphincter function and minimising toxicity. Best outcomes are achieved using a combination of 5-fluorouracil, mitomycin C and radiotherapy. Radiotherapy is best delivered at a minimum dose of 50.4 Gy in 28 fractions over five and a half weeks, initially given in a multifield technique to include the lower pelvis and inguinal nodes with later field reductions to focus on the primary tumour.[23] Using this approach, 3-year overall survival of 75% has recently been reported. Higher doses (upto 70 Gy) have been assessed for larger tumours without significant demonstrable benefit. A gap in treatment was formerly advocated to reduce toxicity and allow assessment of treatment response but is no longer advocated due to recent evidence indicating a negative impact on survival.[23,24]

Radiotherapy alone may be considered for early tumours; however, long-term follow-up data suggest better locoregional control (25% reduction in locoregional relapse) and a 12% risk reduction of dying from anal cancer with combined therapy.[25]

Cisplatin has been compared to mitomycin C in combination with fluorouracil and radiotherapy and been shown to have reduced haematological toxicity; however, it appears to have no advantage with respect to disease-free survival and it may be associated with an increased rate of colostomy formation.[26]

At present there is no evidence to show a survival benefit for neoadjuvant chemotherapy prior to chemoradiotherapy, or for the addition of consolidation chemotherapy.

Factors that negatively impact upon survival include lymph node involvement, large (> 5 cm) tumour diameter and male sex.[27] Local relapse following definitive chemoradiotherapy is significantly more common in HIV-positive patients, and this group is also more likely to develop acute toxicity reactions.[28] Numerous biomarkers have been assessed as potential prognostic factors in anal SCC but none have been shown consistently to predict outcome.

Construction of a defunctioning stoma before therapy in order to manage local symptoms, such as incontinence or fistulation is necessary in approximately 13% of patients.[29] Patients with larger tumours are more likely to require a stoma,[27] although this will be necessary in upto one-third of patients.[30] It is noteworthy that only one-fifth of patients subsequently have their stoma reversed due

> **Key Point**
>
> Combination of 5-fluorouracil, mitomycin C and radiotherapy is the standard therapy for SCC of the anal canal.

to a combination of factors including disease progression, predicted poor functional outcome and persistent fistula.[29]

Management of Inguinal Nodes

Inguinal node disease is treated with chemoradiotherapy as for the treatment of the primary tumour with an additional boost of radiotherapy to the inguinal area. Formal lymphadenectomy may be considered for patients with residual or recurrent disease after chemoradiotherapy. For patients staged node negative, there is no clear consensus on the best management of the inguinal nodes. In patients with early tumours, observation alone seems to be appropriate. In those with more locally advanced disease, prophylactic groin irradiation may be considered; however, any benefit must be balanced with the significant risk of associated morbidity.[31]

Treatment of Recurrent Disease

Persistent or recurrent disease is seen in approximately one-quarter of patients following chemoradiotherapy.[32] Having once been the mainstay of treatment, abdominoperineal excision (APE) is now reserved for patients with recurrence. Salvage APE is associated with 5-year survival in the order of 40–60%.[33-35] Outcomes are worse in patients with positive margins following APE.[36,37] Upto 60% of patients will develop perineal wound problems following APE, and flap reconstruction of the perineum should be considered. In this setting the vertical rectus abdominis myocutaneous (VRAM) flap has been shown to reduce perineal wound complications (27% vs 49%) and healing time, without impacting on overall survival (58% vs 54% 5-year survival) or long-term morbidity.[38]

> **Key Point**
>
> Persistent or recurrent SCC of the anus should be treated by APE. Myocutaneous flap reconstruction reduces the rate of perineal wound problems.

Treatment of Uncommon Anal Tumours

Adenocarcinoma of the anal canal arises from the anal glands and must be distinguished from the more common squamous tumours of different morphologies. Wide local excision is associated with high recurrence rates, and patients should be considered for APE. Five-year survival in the order of 60% has been reported following radical surgery. The value of adjuvant or neoadjuvant radiotherapy in this setting is unclear.[39,40]

Outcomes in patients with melanoma of the anal canal are universally poor; radical surgery gives no survival advantage over local excision.

Paget's disease characteristically presents as an eczematous perianal rash, and the diagnosis is confirmed by the identification of typical Paget cells at histopathological examination. Patients should undergo colonoscopy to exclude a synchronous colorectal cancer. In the absence of invasive disease, treatment is by wide local excision, which should include 1 cm margin of healthy tissue. A split-thickness skin graft, cutaneous flap or a myocutaneous flap may be needed to achieve wound closure. Topical imiquimod has been shown to cause regression of perianal Paget's and may be considered in patients with recurrent disease. Careful follow-up is necessary due to greater than 50% risk of disease recurrence. The presence of invasive disease mandates APE.

Key Points

1. Anal cancer is more common in individuals with risk factors including a history of immunosuppression, HPV infection, smoking, anal dysplasia and in MSM.
2. Squamous cell carcinoma of the anal canal must be distinguished from that of the anal margin as the staging, treatment and prognosis differ according to the site.
3. Staging of the patient with anal cancer should include examination under anaesthesia, CT of thorax/abdomen/pelvis and MRI of pelvis. PET/CT is increasingly useful in the initial staging, particularly for the identification of nodal disease.
4. Patients with focal high-grade dysplasia should undergo surgical excision; those with multifocal disease should undergo excision of symptomatic lesions alone.
5. Combination of 5-fluorouracil, mitomycin C and radiotherapy is the standard therapy for SCC of the anal canal.
6. Persistent or recurrent SCC of the anus should be treated by APE. Myocutaneous flap reconstruction reduces the rate of perineal wound problems.

REFERENCES

1. Faivre J, Trama A, De Angelis R, et al. Incidence, prevalence and survival of patients with rare epithelial digestive cancers diagnosed in Europe in 1995-2002. Eur J Cancer. 2012;48(10):1417-24.
2. Hoots BE, Palefsky JM, Pimenta JM, et al. Human papillomavirus type distribution in anal cancer and anal intraepithelial lesions. Int J Cancer. 2009;124(10):2375-83.
3. Machalek DA, Poynten M, Jin F, et al. Anal human papillomavirus infection and associated neoplastic lesions in men who have sex with men: a systematic review and meta-analysis. Lancet Oncol. 2012;13(5):487-500.
4. Blomberg M, Friis S, Munk C, et al. Genital warts and risk of cancer: a danish study of nearly 50,000 patients with genital warts. J Infect Dis. 2012;205(10):1544-53.
5. Silverberg MJ, Lau B, Justice AC, et al. Risk of anal cancer in HIV-infected and HIV-uninfected individuals in North America. Clin Infect Dis. 2012;54(7):1026-34.
6. Nordenvall C, Nilsson PJ, Ye W, et al. Smoking, snus use and risk of right- and left-sided colon, rectal and anal cancer: a 37-year follow-up study. Int J Cancer. 2011;128(1):157-65.
7. Linam JM, Chand RR, Broudy VC, et al. Evaluation of the impact of HIV serostatus, tobacco smoking and CD4 counts on epidermoid anal cancer survival. Int J STD AIDS. 2012;23(2):77-82.
8. Ramamoorthy S, Luo L, Luo E, et al. Tobacco smoking and risk of recurrence for squamous cell cancer of the anus. Cancer Detect Prev. 2008;32(2):116-20.
9. Scholefield JH, Harris D, Radcliffe A. Guidelines for management of anal intraepithelial neoplasia. Colorectal Dis. 2011;13 Suppl 1:3-10.

10. Palefsky JM, Giuliano AR, Goldstone S, et al. HPV vaccine against anal HPV infection and anal intraepithelial neoplasia. N Engl J Med. 2011;365(17):1576-85.
11. Darragh TM, Winkler B. Anal cancer and cervical cancer screening: key differences. Cancer Cytopathol. 2011;119(1):5-19.
12. Bhuva NJ, Glynne-Jones R, Sonoda L, et al. To PET or not to PET? That is the question. Staging in anal cancer. Ann Oncol. 2012;23(8):2078-82 (Epub ahead of print).
13. Wells IT, Fox BM. PET/CT in anal cancer - is it worth doing? Clin Radiol. 2012;67(6):535-40.
14. Mistrangelo M, Pelosi E, Bello M, et al. Comparison of positron emission tomography scanning and sentinel node biopsy in the detection of inguinal node metastases in patients with anal cancer. Int J Radiat Oncol Biol Phys. 2010;77(1):73-8.
15. Benson AB, Arnoletti JP, Bekaii-Saab T, et al. Anal carcinoma, Version 2.2012: featured updates to the NCCN guidelines. J Natl Compr Canc Netw. 2012;10(4):449-54.
16. Parikh J, Shaw A, Grant LA, et al. Anal carcinomas: the role of endoanal ultrasound and magnetic resonance imaging in staging, response evaluation and follow-up. Eur Radiol. 2011;21(4):776-85.
17. Glynne-Jones R, Northover JM, Cervantes A. Anal cancer: ESMO Clinical Practice Guidelines for diagnosis, treatment and follow-up. Ann Oncol. 2010;21 Suppl 5:v87-92.
18. Renehan AG, O'Dwyer ST. Initial management through the anal cancer multidisciplinary team meeting. Colorectal Dis. 2011;13 Suppl 1:21-8.
19. Damin DC, Rosito MA, Schwartsmann G. Sentinel lymph node in carcinoma of the anal canal: a review. Eur J Surg Oncol. 2006;32(3):247-52.
20. Brown SR, Skinner P, Tidy J, et al. Outcome after surgical resection for high-grade anal intraepithelial neoplasia (Bowen's disease). Br J Surg. 1999;86(8):1063-6.
21. Fox PA, Nathan M, Francis N, et al. A double-blind, randomized controlled trial of the use of imiquimod cream for the treatment of anal canal high-grade anal intraepithelial neoplasia in HIV-positive MSM on HAART, with long-term follow-up data including the use of open-label imiquimod. AIDS. 2010;24(15):2331-5.
22. Khanfir K, Ozsahin M, Bieri S, et al. Patterns of failure and outcome in patients with carcinoma of the anal margin. Ann Surg Oncol. 2008;15(4):1092-8.
23. Kronfli M, Glynne-Jones R. Chemoradiotherapy in anal cancer. Colorectal Dis. 2011;13 Suppl 1:33-8.
24. Glynne-Jones R, Sebag-Montefiore D, Adams R, et al. "Mind the gap"—the impact of variations in the duration of the treatment gap and overall treatment time in the first UK Anal Cancer Trial (ACT I). Int J Radiat Oncol Biol Phys. 2011;81(5):1488-94.
25. Northover J, Glynne-Jones R, Sebag-Montefiore D, et al. Chemoradiation for the treatment of epidermoid anal cancer: 13-year follow-up of the first randomised UKCCCR Anal Cancer Trial (ACT I). Br J Cancer. 2010;102(7):1123-8.
26. Ajani JA, Winter KA, Gunderson LL, et al. Fluorouracil, mitomycin, and radiotherapy vs fluorouracil, cisplatin, and radiotherapy for carcinoma of the anal canal: a randomized controlled trial. JAMA. 2008;299(16):1914-21.
27. Ajani JA, Winter KA, Gunderson LL, et al. US intergroup anal carcinoma trial: tumor diameter predicts for colostomy. J Clin Oncol. 2009;27(7):1116-21.
28. Oehler-Janne C, Huguet F, Provencher S, et al. HIV-specific differences in outcome of squamous cell carcinoma of the anal canal: a multicentric cohort study

of HIV-positive patients receiving highly active antiretroviral therapy. J Clin Oncol. 2008;26(15):2550-7.

29. Cooper R, Mason M, Finan P, et al. Defunctioning stomas prior to chemoradiation for anal cancer are usually permanent. Colorectal Dis. 2012;14(1):87-91.

30. Sunesen KG, Norgaard M, Lundby L, et al. Cause-specific colostomy rates after radiotherapy for anal cancer: a Danish multicentre cohort study. J Clin Oncol. 2011;29(26):3535-40.

31. Branagan G. Staging and management of inguinal nodes. Colorectal Dis. 2011;13 Suppl 1:29-32.

32. Bentzen AG, Guren MG, Wanderas EH, et al. Chemoradiotherapy of anal carcinoma: survival and recurrence in an unselected national cohort. Int J Radiat Oncol Biol Phys. 2012;83(2):e173-80.

33. Mariani P, Ghanneme A, De la Rochefordiere A, et al. Abdominoperineal resection for anal cancer. Dis Colon Rectum. 2008;51(10):1495-501.

34. Nilsson PJ, Svensson C, Goldman S, et al. Salvage abdominoperineal resection in anal epidermoid cancer. Br J Surg. 2002;89(11):1425-9.

35. Mullen JT, Rodriguez-Bigas MA, Chang GJ, et al. Results of surgical salvage after failed chemoradiation therapy for epidermoid carcinoma of the anal canal. Ann Surg Oncol. 2007;14(2):478-83.

36. Eeson G, Foo M, Harrow S, et al. Outcomes of salvage surgery for epidermoid carcinoma of the anus following failed combined modality treatment. Am J Surg. 2011;201(5): 628-33.

37. Sunesen KG, Buntzen S, Tei T, et al. Perineal healing and survival after anal cancer salvage surgery: 10-year experience with primary perineal reconstruction using the vertical rectus abdominis myocutaneous (VRAM) flap. Ann Surg Oncol. 2009;16(1):68-77.

38. Lefevre JH, Parc Y, Kerneis S, et al. Abdomino-perineal resection for anal cancer: impact of a vertical rectus abdominis myocutaneus flap on survival, recurrence, morbidity, and wound healing. Ann Surg. 2009;250(5):707-11.

39. Chang GJ, Gonzalez RJ, Skibber JM, et al. A twenty-year experience with adenocarcinoma of the anal canal. Dis Colon Rectum. 2009;52(8):1375-80.

40. Kounalakis N, Artinyan A, Smith D, et al. Abdominal perineal resection improves survival for nonmetastatic adenocarcinoma of the anal canal. Ann Surg Oncol. 2009;16(5):1310-5.

11 | Intraoperative Radiotherapy in the Management of Locally Advanced and Recurrent Rectal Cancer

Mirnezami R, S Ramkumar, Bateman AR,
Mirnezami AH

BACKGROUND

Colorectal cancer is a major public health issue and represents the second most common cause of cancer-related death in Western societies.[1] In 2009, there were 41,142 new cases of colorectal cancer diagnosed in the UK, of which 64% were primary colonic and 36% were primary rectal tumours.[2] Despite refinements in operative technique, and the widespread adoption of combined-modality treatment (CMT), 5-year survival for colorectal cancer remains at below 60% in most European countries.[3]

Rectal cancer (RC) in particular has a well-established tendency to recur locally, and external beam radiotherapy (EBRT) in combination with chemotherapy has been shown to reduce the risk of both local and distant disease relapse in this setting.[4] Nevertheless, locally advanced rectal cancer (LARC) and locally recurrent rectal cancer (LRRC) continue to present significant therapeutic challenges despite these improvements; LARC is present in approximately 6–14% of all RC cases,[5] and it is estimated that upto 40% of patients with LARC undergoing curative-intent resection will experience local recurrence.[6] In cases of LRRC, the scope for re-irradiation is limited by healthy radiosensitive surrounding viscera, and surgical resection is technically demanding owing to disrupted anatomical planes and frequent involvement of the bony pelvis, which make R0 resection more challenging.[7] Aggressive local control (LC) represents the best chance of improved survival under these circumstances and intraoperative radiotherapy (IORT) has emerged as a potentially valuable treatment modality in the management of these most challenging cases. A number of studies have found that the addition of IORT to conventional CMT strategies for LARC and LRRC can lead to improved LC and survival, although this has not been a universal finding. Here we summarise the available literature on the application of IORT in LARC and LRRC with emphasis on rationale, currently available techniques and long-term oncological outcomes.

RATIONALE

Radiotherapy is firmly established as a key component in the multi-modality management of RC. It is acknowledged that in RC, as with other radiosensitive tumours, tumoricidal effects of radiotherapy are enhanced by increased dose of radiotherapy.[8] Thus, historically, at each period of time when optimisation of techniques has allowed delivery of higher doses of radiation, parallel improvements in LC and survival have also been observed.[9,10] Beyond a certain threshold, however, the radiation tolerance of healthy adjacent structures is exceeded and any potential benefits of radiation are counteracted by unwanted toxicity. To address this limitation, radiation oncologists have employed a number of strategies to improve dose distribution to target areas relative to healthy surrounding tissues. These approaches have included intensity-modulated radiotherapy (IMRT), interstitial brachytherapy and radiosensitisers. Each technique has sought to maximise delivery of radiation to discrete targets whilst simultaneously minimising inadvertent irradiation of healthy surrounding tissues or viscera. Intraoperative radiotherapy represents another approach designed to achieve this aim; IORT is defined as the targeted delivery of radiation to an incompletely resected tumour or tumour bed during surgical resection.[11] This approach allows precise delivery of a single, large fraction of radiation directly to high recurrence-risk anatomical areas, whilst at the same time shielding healthy adjacent viscera.[11] In theory, IORT offers several advantages in the treatment of locally advanced or recurrent CRC. Foremost, is displacement and shielding of adjacent tissue, combined with precise delivery of radiation to the area considered to be at greatest risk for recurrence. Whilst the administered dose is smaller than that delivered with conventional EBRT regimes, the biological effectiveness of a single fraction of IORT is equivalent to two to three times that of conventional EBRT.[10,12] Thus 20 Gy delivered by IORT is estimated to provide the cancer cell-killing effect of 60 Gy provided by conventional EBRT.[10] Additionally, as the radiation dose required for any given degree of tumour control increases with tumour bulk, IORT to any residual tumour after maximal surgical resection is likely to be more effective than conventional fractionated EBRT given to a substantially larger tumour mass prior to surgery.

A more theoretical benefit from IORT stems from the comparatively higher oxygen concentrations present when IORT is delivered. Rectal tumours, like all solid organ malignancies, are subject to significant degrees of intra-tumoral hypoxia as a consequence of unrestrained proliferation

Key Points

- Beyond a certain threshold, the beneficial effect of increasing the dose of external beam irradiation is offset by unwanted toxicity to healthy adjacent viscera. Intra-operative radiotherapy represents one way of circumventing this problem.

- IORT allows targeted delivery of radiation to at-risk target areas identified after surgical resection, whilst simultaneously allowing shielding of adjacent structures.

and impaired or ineffective microvasculature, and severe hypoxia and even anoxia have been noted in both experimental and human cancers. A hypoxic tumour microenvironment has long been associated with increased radiotherapy resistance in tumour cells and the molecular mechanisms behind this are increasingly laid bare.[13-18] This body of research strongly supports the notion that tumour cells irradiated in air show an upto threefold increase in radiosensitivity compared to cells irradiated under hypoxic or anoxic conditions. Thus, for all the reasons outlined above, the application of IORT to difficult and advanced solid organ malignancies is an attractive concept, and seems likely to work synergistically with surgical resection.

TECHNIQUES

Intraoperative radiation in the treatment of LARC and LRRC is delivered using either an electron-based device (IOERT) or by high dose-rate brachytherapy (HDR-IORT).[12] With IOERT, delivery of radiation relies on the emission of high-energy electrons from a linear accelerator, with transmission of the electron beam through a rigid conical applicator. HDR-IORT relies on gamma-emitting radioisotopes [most commonly iridium-92 (^{92}Ir)] that are delivered through hollow catheters to a flexible applicator pad. Each technique has strengths and limitations; treatment and procedure times are generally reduced with IOERT compared with HDR-IORT. In addition IOERT allows the amplitude of electron energy delivered to be varied, thus both deep and superficial areas can be irradiated with this technique.[12] With HDR-IORT, the maximal depth of irradiation is 0.5 cm; however, this disadvantage is offset by the ability to customise the shape of the flexible HDR-IORT applicator, making it highly advantageous for use in curved anatomical spaces such as the pelvis.[10]

The dose of IORT administered is dependent on a number of factors including the volume of residual tumour left behind after maximal surgical resection and whether the patient has previously been treated with EBRT. In the studies presented here, IORT doses range from 7.5 to 25 Gy and 7.5 to 30 Gy for LARC and LRRC, respectively. Doses are typically increased incrementally according to the volume of predicted residual disease after resection (R0 > R1 > R2).[8]

Key Points

- IORT can be delivered using either an electron-based device (IOERT) or by high dose-rate brachytherapy (HDR-IORT).

- With IOERT, procedure times are shorter and the effective depth of irradiation can be varied, whilst the advantage of HDR-IORT is the flexible nature of the applicator pad for use in the pelvis.

- Dosing is dependent on several factors including extent of residual tumour after resection and anticipated radiation tolerance in previously irradiated fields.

ONCOLOGICAL OUTCOMES

Locally Advanced Rectal Cancer

A summary of studies with outcome data for patients with LARC receiving IORT as a component of treatment has been provided in Table 11.1. These studies are largely comprised of single-institution case series, although more recently the results of a large multinational European study and two randomised-controlled trials (RCT) have also been published assessing the impact of IORT in the management of LARC.[19-21] A consistent observation in the literature is the extent of variability in the definition of 'LARC', and this is a source of considerable between-study heterogeneity. The definition of 'locally advanced' in the studies presented ranges from lymph node positive cancers (T1–3)[19,20,22-24] to cases of definitive tumour infiltration to adjacent structures or viscera.[25,26]

TABLE 11.1: Local control and survival after IORT for LARC

Author, Year	N	Resection margin	5-year LC (%)	5-year OS (%)	5-year DFS (%)
Willett et al, 1991[27]	42	R0 R1 R2	88 69 50	—	53 47 17
Huber et al, 1996[28]	38	R0/R1/R2	T3 (84) T4 (90)	28†	—
Nakfoor et al, 1998[29]	73	R0 R1/R2	89 65	—	63 32
Mannaerts et al, 2000[25]	38	R0/R1/R2	82*	72*	65*
Ratto et al, 2003[22]	19	—	91	61	47
Sadahiro et al, 2004[30]	99	—	98	79	71
Nuyttens et al, 2004[31]	18	—	81*	61	—
Diaz-Gonzalez et al, 2006[32]	115	—	94*	74*	74*
Krempien et al, 2006[23]	210	R0 R1/R2	93 77	74 55	68 0
Ferenschild et al, 2006[33]	30	R0 R1/R2	72 58	66 38	—
Roeder et al, 2007[24]	243	R0 R1/R2	94 72	—	—
Masaki et al, 2008[19]	19	—	95	64	60
Mathis et al, 2008[26]	146‡	R0/R1/R2	86	52	43
Valentini et al, 2009[34]	29	R0	100	—	—
Kusters et al, 2010[21]	605	R0/R1/R2	88	67	—
Dubois et al, 2011[20]	68	—	92	77	62

† Overall figures provided by authors for T3 and T4 tumours
* 3-year figures provided by authors
‡ Includes 39 cases of locally advanced colon cancer
Abbreviations: LC: Local control; OS: Overall survival; DFS: Disease-free survival

The largest series to date is a multinational European study reporting outcome data on 605 patients treated with CMT including IORT at four tertiary-referral cancer centres. Five-year local recurrence, overall and disease-free survival were 12%, 67% and 74%, respectively, and these figures compare favourably to the results of contemporary series where IORT has not been incorporated.[21] In addition, a key finding in this study was that 55% of patients with microscopic positive resection margins (R1) remained free of local recurrence at five years, supporting the notion that IORT may eradicate any remaining tumour cells after an R1 resection, offsetting the frequently poor prognosis that this finding confers.

Comparative outcome data for IORT versus non-IORT containing treatment strategies is available from a limited number of studies. In 2006, Ferenschild and colleagues reported outcomes on 123 patients undergoing preoperative EBRT followed by surgery for LARC.[33] Of patients who underwent complete (R0) resection (n=104) 82% (85/104) received no IORT and the remaining 18% (19/104) received a 10 Gy boost of IORT using HDR brachytherapy. No significant difference was observed in LC or survival between these two groups. However, the authors also analysed the impact of IORT in cases where R0 resection was not achieved; in patients who underwent incomplete resection (n=19) 42% (8/19) received no IORT and 58% (11/19) received a single 10 Gy boost to the tumour bed; IORT was found to significantly improve 5-year LC (58% vs 0%) and overall survival (38% vs 0%) in patients undergoing R1/R2 resection. However, it remains unclear whether IORT leads to improved LC after R0 resection; as contrary to the findings of Ferenschild et al, a number of studies have found this to be improved even after complete resection.[22,27,34]

Two recent RCTs have evaluated the impact of IORT[19,20] and neither reported any improvement in LC nor survival compared with conventional treatment approaches. Masaki et al randomised patients with LARC to surgery and IORT (n=19) or surgery alone (n=22). Whilst they observed no significant difference in oncological outcome between the two groups, the small sample size and the inclusion of patients with T1/T2 disease are significant limitations with this study. In a more recent RCT, Dubois et al compared outcomes in 73 patients undergoing surgery and IORT with 69 patients having surgery alone.[20] No significant difference was observed in LC or survival. However, these findings should be interpreted with caution as the high reported rate of 5-year LC in both treatment arms (92% and 93%, respectively for IORT vs no IORT) would suggest that a majority of patients underwent R0 resection, potentially counter-acting any benefit with IORT.

> **Key Point**
>
> A number of studies have reported improved local control with IORT in the management of LARC and most studies have suggested that this benefit is especially significant in the context of incomplete tumour resection. More evidence is needed as in some studies IORT has been shown to improve LC even after R0 resection.

Locally Recurrent Rectal Cancer

A summary of studies with oncological outcome data for IORT in the treatment of LRRC including a total of 933 patients has been provided in Table 11.2. Wiig and co-workers evaluated outcomes in 107 patients with LRRC of whom 59 received IORT as a component of treatment. For patients undergoing R0 resection, 5-year survival was equivalent at around 60% in both IORT and non-IORT treatment groups. However, the authors noted significantly improved LC amongst patients receiving IORT (50% vs 30% at 5 years).[35] Similar findings have been reported in a number of other studies.

TABLE 11.2: Local control and survival after IORT for LRRC

Author, Year	N	Resection margin	5-year LC (%)	5-year OS (%)	5-year DFS (%)
Willett et al, 1991[36]	30	R0 R1/R2	62 18	—	54 6
Eble et al, 1998[37]	31	R0 R1/R2	79 65	—	71 29
Valentini et al, 1999[38]	11	—	80	41	19
Lindel et al, 2001[39]	49	R0 R1/R2	56 17	46 14	32 8
Wiig et al, 2002[35]	59	R0/R1/R2	44	30	—
Pezner et al, 2002[40]	15φ	R0/R1/R2	25*	29*	—
Shoup et al, 2002[41]	100	R0/R1/R2	—	—	22
Hashiguchi et al, 2003[42]	39§	R0/R1/R2 R0	— 24	13 35	— 24
Nuyttens et al, 2004[31]	19	—	48	34	—
Dresen et al, 2008[43]	147	R0 R1 R2	75* 29* 29*	59* 27* 24*	—
Vermaas et al, 2008[44]	11	R0/R1/R2	27*	51*	—
Haddock et al, 2011[45]	607†	R0 R1 R2	79 68ϖ	46 27 16	—

φ Includes two cases of locally recurrence colon cancer
* 3-year figures provided by authors
§ Includes three cases of locally recurrent colon cancer
† Includes 182 cases of locally recurrent colon cancer
ϖ Combined data for R1/R2 resections
Abbreviations: LC: Local control; OS: Overall survival; DFS: Disease-free survival

To date, the largest series assessing the impact of CMT incorporating IORT in LRRC has been reported by the Mayo Clinic.[45] This study included 607 patients undergoing treatment for local recurrence over a 27-year period, and all cases received IORT. LRRC represented 427 cases (70%), whilst the remainders were colonic recurrences. Overall 5- and 10-year survivals were 30% and 16%, respectively with 5-year survival as high as

46% in patients undergoing R0 resection. Of note, excellent long-term oncological outcomes were found in 224 R1 and 156 R2 resections receiving IORT,

with 5-year survival of 27% and 16% respectively, and an outstanding 5-year rate of LC of 68%.

SUMMARY AND FUTURE DIRECTIONS

Intraoperative radiotherapy represents a highly specialised form of focused radiotherapy which permits treatment intensification to the cancer-bed and areas at-risk, whilst limiting the deleterious effects of radiotherapy on normal tissue. The studies summarised here suggest that an aggressive multi-modal approach, encompassing IORT where appropriate, may offer the optimal management in cases of LARC and LRRC.

A number of questions still remain however; the exact dose and depth of penetration for maximal efficacy in different tumour subtypes and anatomical locations within the pelvis remains unclear. In addition, an important question to address is whether delivery of IORT may facilitate an increase in preservation of organs which would otherwise have been sacrificed surgically to prevent a close or microscopically involved margin, and whether IORT can truly compensate for a positive resection margin. In the future,

Key Points

1. Beyond a certain threshold, the beneficial effect of increasing the dose of external beam irradiation is offset by unwanted toxicity to healthy adjacent viscera. Intra-operative radiotherapy represents one way of circumventing this problem.

2. IORT allows targeted delivery of radiation to at-risk target areas identified after surgical resection, whilst simultaneously allowing shielding of adjacent structures.

3. IORT can be delivered using either an electron-based device (IOERT) or by high dose-rate brachytherapy (HDR-IORT).

4. With IOERT, procedure times are shorter and the effective depth of irradiation can be varied, whilst the advantage of HDR-IORT is the flexible nature of the applicator pad for use in the pelvis.

5. Dosing is dependent on several factors including extent of residual tumour after resection and anticipated radiation tolerance in previously irradiated fields.

6. A number of studies have reported improved local control with IORT in the management of LARC and most studies have suggested that this benefit is especially significant in the context of incomplete tumour resection. More evidence is needed as in some studies IORT has been shown to improve LC even after R0 resection.

7. Although level 1 evidence is lacking, inclusion of IORT into established CMT regimes in LRRC appears to improve local control.

high-number multi-institutional studies with limited heterogeneity in the indication for surgical intervention (i.e. LARC or LRRC), type of resection performed (R0 or R1/R2), and the application of adjuvant treatments, may better enable clarification of the independent contribution of IORT to the treatment of complex RC.

REFERENCES

1. Cunningham D, Atkin W, Lenz HJ, et al. Colorectal cancer. Lancet. 2010;375(9719):1030-47.
2. Cancer Research UK. Bowel cancer—UK incidence statistics. 2012.
3. Verdecchia A, Francisci S, Brenner H, et al. Recent cancer survival in Europe: a 2000−02 period analysis of EUROCARE-4 data. Lancet Oncol. 2007;8(9):784-96.
4. Bosset JF, Calais G, Mineur L, et al. Enhanced tumorocidal effect of chemotherapy with preoperative radiotherapy for rectal cancer: preliminary results—EORTC 22921. J Clin Oncol. 2005;23(24):5620-7.
5. Luna-Perez P, Delgado S, Labastida S, et al. Patterns of recurrence following pelvic exenteration and external radiotherapy for locally advanced primary rectal adenocarcinoma. Ann Surg Oncol. 1996;3(6):526-33.
6. Harrison LB, Minsky BD, Enker WE, et al. High dose rate intraoperative radiation therapy (HDR-IORT) as part of the management strategy for locally advanced primary and recurrent rectal cancer. Int J Radiat Oncol Biol Phys. 1998;42(2):325-30.
7. Austin KK, Solomon MJ. Pelvic exenteration with en bloc iliac vessel resection for lateral pelvic wall involvement. Dis Colon Rectum. 2009;52(7):1223-33.
8. Calvo FA, Meirino RM, Orecchia R. Intraoperative radiation therapy first part: rationale and techniques. Crit Rev Oncol Hematol. 2006;59(2):106-15.
9. Gunderson LL, Shipley WU, Suit HD, et al. Intraoperative irradiation: a pilot study combining external beam photons with "boost" dose intraoperative electrons. Cancer. 1982;49(11):2259-66.
10. Willett CG, Czito BG, Tyler DS. Intraoperative radiation therapy. J Clin Oncol. 2007;25(8):971-7.
11. Gunderson LL. Rationale for and results of intraoperative radiation therapy. Cancer. 1994;74(2):537-41.
12. Skandarajah AR, Lynch AC, Mackay JR, et al. The role of intraoperative radiotherapy in solid tumors. Ann Surg Oncol. 2009;16(3):735-44.
13. Palcic B, Skarsgard LD. Reduced oxygen enhancement ratio at low doses of ionizing radiation. Radiat Res. 1984;100(2):328-39.
14. Alper T, Howard-Flanders P. Role of oxygen in modifying the radiosensitivity of *E. coli* B. Nature. 1956;178(4540):978-9.
15. Hockel M, Schlenger K, Mitze M, et al. Hypoxia and radiation response in human tumors. Semin Radiat Oncol. 1996;6(1):3-9.
16. Wang JZ, Li XA, Mayr NA. Dose escalation to combat hypoxia in prostate cancer: a radiobiological study on clinical data. Br J Radiol. 2006;79(947):905-11.
17. Chan N, Koritzinsky M, Zhao H, et al. Chronic hypoxia decreases synthesis of homologous recombination proteins to offset chemoresistance and radioresistance. Cancer Res. 2008;68(2):605-14.
18. Dietz DW, Dehdashti F, Grigsby PW, et al. Tumor hypoxia detected by positron emission tomography with 60Cu-ATSM as a predictor of response and survival in patients undergoing neoadjuvant chemoradiotherapy for rectal carcinoma: a pilot study. Dis Colon Rectum. 2008;51(11):1641-8.
19. Masaki T, Takayama M, Matsuoka H, et al. Intraoperative radiotherapy for oncological and function-preserving surgery in patients with advanced lower rectal cancer. Langenbecks Arch Surg. 2008;393(2):173-80.

20. Dubois JB, Bussieres E, Richaud P, et al. Intra-operative radiotherapy of rectal cancer: results of the French multi-institutional randomized study. Radiother Oncol. 2011;98(3):298-303.
21. Kusters M, Valentini V, Calvo FA, et al. Results of European pooled analysis of IORT-containing multimodality treatment for locally advanced rectal cancer: adjuvant chemotherapy prevents local recurrence rather than distant metastases. Ann Oncol. 2010;21(6):1279-84.
22. Ratto C, Valentini V, Morganti AG, et al. Combined-modality therapy in locally advanced primary rectal cancer. Dis Colon Rectum. 2003;46(1):59-67.
23. Krempien R, Roeder F, Oertel S, et al. Long-term results of intraoperative presacral electron boost radiotherapy (IOERT) in combination with total mesorectal excision (TME) and chemoradiation in patients with locally advanced rectal cancer. Int J Radiat Oncol Biol Phys. 2006;66(4):1143-51.
24. Roeder F, Treiber M, Oertel S, et al. Patterns of failure and local control after intraoperative electron boost radiotherapy to the presacral space in combination with total mesorectal excision in patients with locally advanced rectal cancer. Int J Radiat Oncol Biol Phys. 2007;67(5):1381-8.
25. Mannaerts GH, Martijn H, Crommelin MA, et al. Feasibility and first results of multimodality treatment, combining EBRT, extensive surgery, and IOERT in locally advanced primary rectal cancer. Int J Radiat Oncol Biol Phys. 2000;47(2):425-33.
26. Mathis KL, Nelson H, Pemberton JH, et al. Unresectable colorectal cancer can be cured with multimodality therapy. Ann Surg. 2008;248(4):592-8.
27. Willett CG, Shellito PC, Tepper JE, et al. Intraoperative electron beam radiation therapy for primary locally advanced rectal and rectosigmoid carcinoma. J Clin Oncol. 1991;9(5):843-9.
28. Huber FT, Stepan R, Zimmermann F, et al. Locally advanced rectal cancer: resection and intraoperative radiotherapy using the flab method combined with preoperative or postoperative radiochemotherapy. Dis Colon Rectum. 1996;39(7):774-9.
29. Nakfoor BM, Willett CG, Shellito PC, et al. The impact of 5-fluorouracil and intraoperative electron beam radiation therapy on the outcome of patients with locally advanced primary rectal and rectosigmoid cancer. Ann Surg. 1998;228(2):194-200.
30. Sadahiro S, Suzuki T, Ishikawa K, et al. Preoperative radio/chemo-radiotherapy in combination with intraoperative radiotherapy for T3-4Nx rectal cancer. Eur J Surg Oncol. 2004;30(7):750-8.
31. Nuyttens JJ, Kolkman-Deurloo IK, Vermaas M, et al. High-dose-rate intraoperative radiotherapy for close or positive margins in patients with locally advanced or recurrent rectal cancer. Int J Radiat Oncol Biol Phys. 2004;58(1):106-12.
32. Diaz-Gonzalez JA, Calvo FA, Cortes J, et al. Prognostic factors for disease-free survival in patients with T3-4 or N+ rectal cancer treated with preoperative chemoradiation therapy, surgery, and intraoperative irradiation. Int J Radiat Oncol Biol Phys. 2006;64(4):1122-8.
33. Ferenschild FT, Vermaas M, Nuyttens JJ, et al. Value of intraoperative radiotherapy in locally advanced rectal cancer. Dis Colon Rectum. 2006;49(9):1257-65.
34. Valentini V, Coco C, Rizzo G, et al. Outcomes of clinical T4M0 extra-peritoneal rectal cancer treated with preoperative radiochemotherapy and surgery: a prospective evaluation of a single institutional experience. Surgery. 2009;145(5):486-94.
35. Wiig JN, Tveit KM, Poulsen JP, et al. Preoperative irradiation and surgery for recurrent rectal cancer. Will intraoperative radiotherapy (IORT) be of additional benefit? A prospective study. Radiother Oncol. 2002;62(2):207-13.

36. Willett CG, Shellito PC, Tepper JE, et al. Intraoperative electron beam radiation therapy for recurrent locally advanced rectal or rectosigmoid carcinoma. Cancer. 1991;67(6):1504-8.
37. Eble MJ, Lehnert T, Treiber M, et al. Moderate dose intraoperative and external beam radiotherapy for locally recurrent rectal carcinoma. Radiother Oncol. 1998;49(2):169-74.
38. Valentini V, Morganti AG, De Franco A, et al. Chemoradiation with or without intraoperative radiation therapy in patients with locally recurrent rectal carcinoma: prognostic factors and long-term outcome. Cancer. 1999;86(12):2612-24.
39. Lindel K, Willett CG, Shellito PC, et al. Intraoperative radiation therapy for locally advanced recurrent rectal or rectosigmoid cancer. Radiother Oncol. 2001;58(1):83-7.
40. Pezner RD, Chu DZ, Ellenhorn JD. Intraoperative radiation therapy for patients with recurrent rectal and sigmoid colon cancer in previously irradiated fields. Radiother Oncol. 2002;64(1):47-52.
41. Shoup M, Guillem JG, Alektiar KM, et al. Predictors of survival in recurrent rectal cancer after resection and intraoperative radiotherapy. Dis Colon Rectum. 2002;45(5):585-92.
42. Hashiguchi Y, Sekine T, Kato S, et al. Indicators for surgical resection and intraoperative radiation therapy for pelvic recurrence of colorectal cancer. Dis Colon Rectum. 2003;46(1):31-9.
43. Dresen RC, Gosens MJ, Martijn H, et al. Radical resection after IORT-containing multimodality treatment is the most important determinant for outcome in patients treated for locally recurrent rectal cancer. Ann Surg Oncol. 2008;15(7):1937-47.
44. Vermaas M, Nuyttens JJ, Ferenschild FT, et al. Reirradiation, surgery and IORT for recurrent rectal cancer in previously irradiated patients. Radiother Oncol. 2008;87(3):357-60.
45. Haddock MG, Miller RC, Nelson H, et al. Combined modality therapy including intraoperative electron irradiation for locally recurrent colorectal cancer. Int J Radiat Oncol Biol Phys. 2011;79(1):143-50.

12 | Modern Management of Abdominal Tuberculosis

VK Kapoor

INTRODUCTION

Tuberculosis (TB), also called Koch's disease (Robert Koch discovered the organism in 1882), continues to be prevalent all over the world, although incidence rates are falling globally, except in South-East Asia where they are still stable. In the underdeveloped and developing Third World, the disease persists due to poverty, overcrowding and malnutrition. Transglobal migration and movement of populations are responsible for the resurgence of the disease in the developed Western world. About 10 million new cases of TB occur every year.

MICROBIOLOGY

Human TB is caused by *Mycobacterium tuberculosis*. Tuberculosis occurs in cattle also where it is caused by *M. bovis* which is secreted in milk. Human infection due to *M. bovis* does not occur in countries like India due to universal practice of boiling milk before it is consumed but in countries, where unpasteurised milk and milk products are used, it still continues to occur. Human immunodeficiency virus (HIV) patients are more likely to be infected with atypical mycobacteria, e.g. *M. avium* complex. Mycobacteria are classified as acid-fast bacilli (AFB) and can be detected on smear by Ziehl-Neelsen and auramine-rhodamine fluorescent stain and can be cultured in Lowenstein-Jensen medium or BACTEC 460 TB liquid medium; the latter provides better yield.[1]

PATHOGENESIS

The abdomen is not usually the primary site of involvement in TB. Lung is the primary site of involvement as mycobateria contained in the sputum of an infected patient spread by aerosol. Ingested mycobacteria (either in the swallowed sputum from an active lung lesion or in infected milk) enter the lymphoid tissue in the Peyer's patches in the small intestine where they are taken up by the macrophages which travel to the mesenteric lymph nodes.

The abdomen may also be involved as a result of haematological spread from a primary lesion or secondary to involvement of the genital tract (tubo-ovarian) in women.

IMMUNOLOGY

Tuberculosis is the best example of the interplay between the virulence of the organism and the immunity of the host. In tuberculosis, infection with the organism is not the same as clinical disease. Almost one-third of the World population is infected with the organism but there are only about 15 million active cases. In most patients, the primary focus (in lungs or lymph nodes) does not cause clinical disease and heals by itself but the organism survives, although remaining dormant. Immunocompromised or immunosuppression, e.g. old age, alcoholism, malnutrition, diabetes mellitus, HIV, cancer, end stage renal disease, post-transplant immunosuppression, prolonged steroids use, etc. can result in reactivation of a dormant primary focus so that latent infection becomes active and causes disease.

PATHOLOGY

Commonest site of involvement in TB is lungs (pulmonary TB); extra-pulmonary disease is present in about 15–20% of patients. Common extra-pulmonary sites of involvement are lymph nodes, genitourinary tract and bones and joints followed by the abdomen (accounting for 2–5% of all cases of TB). Extra-pulmonary TB is more frequent in HIV positive patients than in HIV negative.

By definition, abdominal TB includes the involvement of the gastrointestinal (GI) tract, peritoneum and lymph nodes; solid viscera, e.g. liver, spleen and pancreas, can also be rarely involved. The proportion of involvement of these sites differs between medical and surgical series; intestinal lesions being more common in surgical series and peritoneal and nodal lesions being more common in medical reports. Terminal ileum and ileocaecal region are the most common sites of involvement in GI TB, followed by jejunum and colon. Multiple sites of involvement (GI tract, peritoneum and/or lymph nodes) and multiple lesions are the common features. Peritoneal and solid viscera involvement is more common as a part of miliary TB.[2]

Gastrointestinal lesions can be ulcerative, hypertrophic (hyperplastic) or stricturing. Peritoneum TB can be wet (ascitic) type which in turn can be generalised, localised or encysted, or dry (fibrinous, adhesive) type with thick mesentery, rolled up omentum, matted bowel loops and even cocoon (Fig. 12.1) formation.[3] Mesenteric lymph nodes are most commonly involved but periportal peripancreatic and aortocaval lymph nodes can also be involved.

The characteristic histological picture of TB is the presence of epithelioid cell granulomas with lymphocytes and plasma cells with central caseating

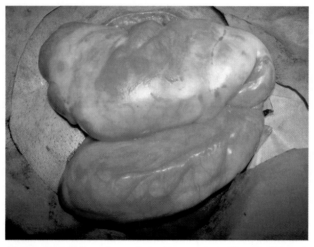

Figure 12.1: Tubercular peritoneal cocoon engulfing small bowel

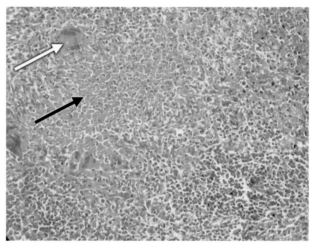

Figure 12.2: Epitheloid cell granulomas with Langhan's giant cells (white arrow) and caseation necrosis (black arrow)

necrosis and Langhan's giant cells (Fig. 12.2). Healing occurs by fibrosis (resulting in strictures in the small intestine) and may be followed by calcification (commonly seen in lymph nodes).

CLINICAL FEATURES

Tuberculosis is a disease of young adults but can occur at any age—in children, peritoneal and lymph node TB is more frequent than GI TB; a large central abdominal nodular lump (tabes mesenterica) is not an uncommon presentation.

Abdominal TB has varied modes of presentation (chronic or subacute, acute-on-chronic and acute) and several methods of presentation (lump, ascites, obstruction, perforation and peritonitis). Symptoms of abdominal TB may be:

- General—fever, night sweats, anorexia and weight loss, failure to thrive (in children), malaise, fatigue, lethargy and lassitude
- Abdominal—pain, distension, bowel disturbances including both diarrhoea (due to ulcerated lesions and malabsorption) and constipation (due to obstruction); *gola* formation (moving ball of wind), borborygmi (audible sounds of exaggerated bowel peristalsis).

A lump may be palpable, most commonly in the right iliac fossa (hypertrophic ileocaecal TB), central abdomen (enlarged mesenteric lymph nodes), ilioinguinal (iliopsoas abscess secondary to spinal TB), upper abdomen (rolled up omentum, omental cake), lower abdomen (tubo-ovarian mass due to associated genital tract TB) or anywhere in the abdomen (colonic hypertrophic TB, matted bowel loops, loculated ascites).

Signs include pallor, malnutrition, wasting and deficiencies; abdominal lump and organomegaly. In peritoneal TB with ascites, abdomen is distended and doughy and is mildly tender.

Symptoms of involvement of other systems, e.g. lungs (cough, haemoptysis and chest pain), lymph nodes (neck, mediastinum), bones and joints, genital tract (oligohypomenorrhoea and amenorrhoea and infertility) may be present. Family history of TB, even if present and known, is very often not disclosed due to the social stigma still attached to the disease.

> **Key Point**
>
> Clinical features of abdominal TB include general symptoms of the disease, and abdominal pain, distension, bowel disturbance, and the presence of a palpable mass or ascites.

UNUSUAL SITES

Oesophagus may be involved secondary to TB in the mediastinal lymph nodes and mimics cancer—fever and painful dysphagia (odynophagia) suggest the diagnosis of TB. Endoscopy reveals ulcers and nodularity (no mass or growth) and contrast study may reveal a sinus or even a fistula (oesophagotracheal or oesophagobronchial). Gastroduodenal TB mimics peptic ulcer disease (PUD) or cancer; fibrotic healing of prepyloric or pyloric TB ulcer may result in pyloric stenosis. Short duration of symptoms, early onset of gastric outlet obstruction, unusual or bizarre endoscopic findings and non-response to standard anti-ulcer treatment should raise the suspicion of TB and warrant repeat endoscopy and biopsy. Multiple or recurrent fistula-in-ano should raise the suspicion of TB. Enlarged TB lymph nodes at the root of small bowel mesentery may cause extrinsic D3-D4 compression; those in the hepatoduodenal ligament can cause portal venous obstruction and portal hypertension[4] or biliary obstruction and obstructive jaundice.

Peripancreatic lymph nodes may mimic a pancreatic mass on imaging.[5] Unsuspected (peritoneal) TB is a common cause of persistent discharging non-healing sinus after laparoscopic surgery. Liver[6] and spleen[7] involvement may be in the form of elevation of hepatic enzymes, organomegaly, micro nodules, tuberculoma or abscess. Tuberculosis of the biliary tract may mimic malignant obstruction.[8]

ACUTE PRESENTATION

Abdominal TB classically has a chronic mode of presentation with history dating to months or even years. In some patients, this long clinical course is interspersed with an acute attack (usually obstruction, sometimes perforation)—acute-on-chronic presentation; rarely, an acute abdomen is the first presentation of abdominal TB.[9]

Intestinal obstruction is common in TB;[10] obstruction can be caused in TB by strictures, hypertrophic lesions and adhesions. Tuberculosis is not an uncommon cause of intestinal obstruction; in another study from India, 52/367 (14%) cases of intestinal obstruction were caused by TB.[11] In tropical countries, TB is the second most common cause of small bowel perforation after typhoid.[12] Perforation occurs at the site of an ulcer, usually proximal to a stricture.[13] Massive lower GI bleed due to TB ulcers is rare. Tuberculosis pancolitis mimicking ulcerative colitis has also been reported. Peritoneal TB can present as acute peritonitis (with no bowel perforation) and acute TB mesenteric lymphadenitis (due to caseation) has also been reported.

Tuberculosis toxaemia is usually seen in patients with miliary (multi-system) TB or sometimes in peritoneal TB. Patient looks ill, has fever, tachycardia, tachypnoea, leucocytosis and elevated CRP.

DIFFERENTIAL DIAGNOSIS

Tuberculosis is a great mimic and can masquerade as many other clinical problems.[14] Abdominal TB (lump and GI bleed with anorexia and weight loss) can mimic intra-abdominal malignancy. Enlarged TB lymph nodes may resemble lymphoma; contrast-enhanced MRI can help to differentiate between the two.[15] Caseating mesenteric lymph nodes may produce a pseudocyst (Fig. 12.3). Tuberculosis tubo-ovarian masses will look like ovarian tumours. Multiple peritoneal and omental tubercles may be difficult to differentiate from peritoneal carcinomatosis which is common in ovary and stomach; tubercles are uniform in size whereas nodules in carcinomatosis are of varying sizes and may show umbilication; serum CA 125 may be high in TB also, but CA 19-9 and CEA are normal.[16,17] In the absence of granulomas, it is impossible to differentiate TB ulcers and strictures from ischaemic lesions.[18] It is important to differentiate between TB ascites and ascites due to cirrhosis as most anti-tubercular therapies (ATTs) are hepatotoxic. Loculated TB ascites may appear like a

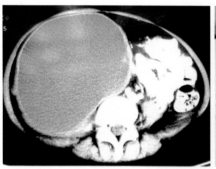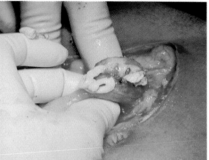

Figure 12.3: CT scan showing large cystic lesion in abdomen; yellow cheesy material coming out of the abdominal cyst—cold abscess

cyst (pancreatic pseudocyst in upper abdomen, mesenteric cyst in central abdomen or ovarian cyst in lower abdomen). Malabsorption of TB has to be differentiated from other common causes, e.g. celiac disease, tropical sprue, immunoproliferative small intestinal disease (IPSID), etc.[19] Abdominal (especially peritoneal, lymph node and solid organ) TB may masquerade as pyrexia of unknown origin (PUO) or unexplained weight loss.

Tuberculosis mimics Crohn's disease not only on imaging but on histopathology also. Diarrhoea, a common feature in Crohn's, is less common in TB; perianal lesions and fistulae (internal and external) of Crohn's are rare in TB; caseating lymph nodes and tubercles are characteristic of TB; strictures in TB are short and annular (cf. long and tubular in Crohn's); TB granulomas are caseating (cf. non-caseating in Crohn's).

INVESTIGATIONS

Anaemia, hypoproteinaemia and hypoalbuminaemia are frequently present due to malnutrition. Raised ESR and elevated CRP are non-specific markers which are of no use in diagnosis but should be obtained before starting ATT as they may be a good marker to assess the response.

Radiology plays an important role in diagnosis of abdominal TB.[20] Chest X-ray, if positive (for pulmonary or pleural TB), is helpful in diagnosis, but a normal chest X-ray does not rule out the diagnosis of abdominal TB. Plain X-rays of the abdomen may show calcified mesenteric lymph nodes, ground glass appearance of ascites, dilated loops with air fluid levels and free air. Barium studies [meal follow through enteroclysis (Fig. 12.4) and enema (Fig. 12.5)] show irritability and hurry (due to mucosal inflammation), flocculation and fragmentation of barium, nodular thickening of mucosal folds, contracted irregular shortened narrowed deformed cone-shaped pulled up caecum, incompetent ileocaecal valve, bowel loops displaced to the periphery with empty centre of the abdomen (due to enlarged lymph nodes) and adherent fixed loops.

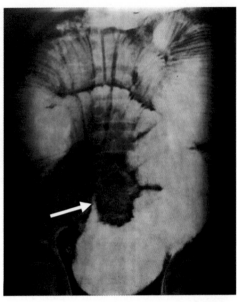

Figure 12.4: Small bowel enema (enteroclysis) showing hugely dilated proximal small bowel loops with a jejunal stricture (arrow)

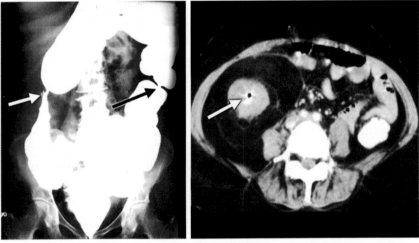

Figure 12.5: Barium enema showing right colon stricture (white arrow), another stricture is seen in left colon also (black arrow); CT scan showing thickened right colon (arrow)

Ultrasonography (US) may show hyperechoic mesenteric thickening (> 15 mm), enlarged mesenteric lymph nodes, ascites, thickened bowel loops and ileocaecal or colonic mass. Computed tomography (CT) shows diffuse (cf. nodular in cancer) mesenteric, omental and peritoneal thickening with stranding, dilated matted bowel loops, enlarged lymph nodes with peripheral rim-like enhancement and hypodense (caseation necrosis) centre[21]

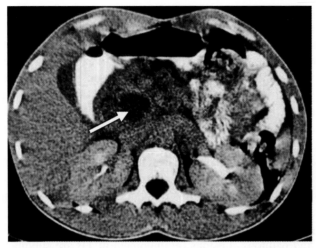

Figure 12.6: CT scan showing large retrogastric lymph node with central necrosis (arrow)

(Fig. 12.6) and adnexal (tubo-ovarian) mass. On PET scan, TB lesions, especially peritoneal and lymph nodes, may have false positive high uptake and may look malignant.[22,23]

Skin tests done with purified protein derivative (PPD) of tuberculin are not helpful, as false positive results are very common due to previous sensitisation by contact and BCG vaccination (which is part of immunisation programme in many countries including India). Serological tests only suggest but do not confirm the diagnosis of TB.

The hallmark of diagnosis of TB anywhere in the body is demonstration of AFB on histology, smear or culture. Yield of AFB in extra-pulmonary TB in general and in abdominal TB in particular is low and a microbiological diagnosis of abdominal TB is difficult in most cases. Acid-fast bacilli are more likely to be present in more virulent forms of abdominal TB, i.e. ascitic type of peritoneal TB and miliary TB; AFB are less likely to be seen in lymph node and GI lesions. In patients with ulcerative GI TB, AFB may be present in gastric aspirate or stool. It is, however, acceptable to diagnose abdominal TB on histopathology alone by demonstration of caseating granulomas. Tissue for microbiological or histopathological diagnosis can be obtained by endoscopy (lower GI or upper GI), US/endoscopic US[24,25]/CT guided fine needle aspiration cytology (FNAC) or laparoscopy. Detection of mycobacterial DNA in tissues by PCR is highly sensitive.[26]

Ascitic fluid in TB is a clear straw-coloured exudate with protein greater than 3 G/L, serum ascites albumin gradient (SAAG) less than 1.1 and cells greater than 1,000/ mL, predominantly lymphocytes. Ascitic fluid adenosine deaminase (ADA) greater than 33 U/L suggests TB;[27,28] but ADA may be normal or even low in TB patients with HIV. Ascitic fluid ADA may also be elevated in malignant ascites.

Demonstration of AFB on Ziehl-Neelsen (ZN) stain of ascitic fluid smear is rare; it was seen in only 1/53 cases.[29] Acid-fast bacilli culture may be positive in upto 20-40% of cases—aspiration of large (about 1 litre) amount of ascitic fluid and its centrifugation increases the yield. In patients with (ascitic) peritoneal TB, percutaneous, laparoscopic or mini-laparotomy peritoneal biopsy provides tissue for diagnosis. Laparoscopy shows thickened hyperemic peritoneum with loss of lustre and tubercles (yellowish-white 2-5 mm soft to firm nodules) on the omentum and parietal and visceral peritoneum.[29,30]

Endoscopy shows submucosal nodules and multiple 2-5 mm discrete transversely placed circumferential superficial (cf. deep in Crohn's disease) mucosal ulcers with sharp but irregular undermined edges; pseudopolyps (as seen in ulcerative colitis) may also be seen. The caecum is rigid contracted shortened and deformed, and the ileocaecal valve is thickened edematous deformed and patulous. Lesions (granulomas) in TB are submucosal—deep (biopsy-on-biopsy) biopsies are required; yield may be better with FNAC. Liver biopsy may reveal the diagnosis in patients with hepatomegaly and those with suspected miliary TB.

Anorectal, colonic and ileocaecal lesions can be seen and biopsied on lower GI endoscopy (ano-procto-sigmoido-colonoscopy). An expert endoscopist can (retrogradely) enter the terminal ileum through the ileocaecal valve and visualise and biopsy the distal ileum. Lesions in oesophagus, stomach and duodenum, although rare, can be accessed easily on upper GI endoscopy. Proximal jejunum can be seen on double balloon enteroscope or push enteroscope. It is the mid small bowel (distal jejunum and proximal ileum) which is inaccessible to endoscopy. Capsule endoscope can visualise the entire small bowel but should be used with caution in patients with suspected TB as it may get arrested at the site of a subclinical stricture; also, it does not offer the opportunity of obtaining tissue for diagnosis.

Therapeutic trial (institution of ATT on clinical and radiological suspicion alone to observe its response) is advocated and practised by many but is not recommended by the author as it may delay the treatment of many other conditions, including cancer, which may mimic abdominal TB even on imaging. Diagnosis of abdominal TB was confirmed in only 46 out of 110 cases in which there was clinical suspicion of TB.[31] Moreover, 4-6 weeks of ATT may alter the histopathology of TB so that later confirmation of diagnosis of TB becomes difficult.

COINFECTION WITH HIV

Many tuberculologists had predicted the eradication of TB[32] but emergence of HIV and AIDS demolished their hopes. The immunosuppression of HIV infection not only promotes reactivation of dormant TB infection (which is quite prevalent) but also predisposes the patient to new TB infection.[33] HIV infection may be present in about $10\%^{34}$ of patients with abdominal TB. HIV patients have a 10% annual risk of developing TB. The dual epidemic of TB and HIV affects an estimated 4 million people worldwide; 20% (400,000) of 2 million TB deaths every year occur in those with TB and HIV.

COEXISTENCE WITH CANCER

In areas and populations where TB is still common, all enlarged lymph nodes in patients with cancer are not necessarily metastatic; they may be harbouring coexisting TB. Tissue diagnosis must be obtained from enlarged lymph nodes by FNAC if this alters the management plan, e.g. administration of neoadjuvant chemoradiotherapy, decision about resectability for cure, extent of lymph node dissection, etc.

ANTITUBERCULAR THERAPY

Most patients with peritoneal, lymph nodes and solid organ TB, and many patients with GI TB can be treated with ATT. All patients with abdominal TB, including those who are operated, should receive a full course of ATT. A combination of drugs is always used to reduce emergence of resistance. Both 6 months (4 drugs for 2 months followed by 2 drugs for 4 months) and 9 months (3 drugs for 3 months followed by 2 drugs for 6 months) courses are equally (99% vs 94%) effective in abdominal TB.[35] Directly observed treatment short course (DOTS) includes supervised administration of drugs 2–3 times a week. Prolonged course of ATT may be required in immuno-suppression. Antitubercular drugs are hepatotoxic—liver function tests should be monitored. Patients should be counselled to complete the course as inadequate treatment is responsible for multidrug resistant (MDR) TB.

The role of steroids in abdominal TB is controversial. By and large, there is no indication for their use in abdominal TB except when abdominal TB is part of miliary TB and patients present with TB toxaemia or have an Addisonian crisis due to bilateral adrenal involvement. In patients with peritoneal TB, especially of ascitic type, addition of steroids to ATT for the first 4–6 weeks may reduce the future risk of formation of adhesions.

SURGERY

Laparoscopy plays an important role in the diagnosis of abdominal TB, especially the ascitic type of peritoneal TB. Diagnostic laparotomy is now rarely indicated for TB as it should be possible to make a diagnosis based on radiology, imaging and endoscopy.

Patients with an acute abdomen (obstruction, perforation and peritonitis) may be found to have unsuspected TB at laparotomy. Intestinal obstruction in TB is usually subacute and settles with conservative management allowing for elective surgery later. Tubercular perforations can be closed, resected (if associated with a distal stricture) or exteriorised (in presence of severe peritonitis).

Indications for elective surgery in TB include doubt in diagnosis, e.g. a lump, where malignancy cannot be ruled out or complications, e.g. recurrent obstruction. Surgical procedures in TB are conservative, e.g. limited resection for ileocaecal mass (Fig. 12.7) but a radical resection, such as right hemicolectomy, should be performed if malignancy cannot be ruled out; strictures can be resected or strictureplasty[36] (Fig. 12.8) can be performed. Bypass procedures are avoided as they may result in a blind loop. Splenectomy may rarely be indicated to treat a TB splenic abscess.

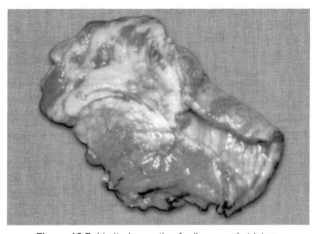

Figure 12.7: Limited resection for ileocaecal stricture

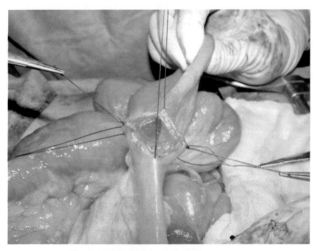

Figure 12.8: Strictureplasty in progress

OUTCOME

Tuberculosis is an infectious disease which should be associated with no or a very low mortality; but it is not so. Tuberculosis causes 2 million deaths every year worldwide, but only $1-3\%$ are caused by abdominal TB. Mortality of abdominal TB is high $(5-10\%)$[11,37,38] in acute presentation, in patients with HIV, in MDR TB and in patients with miliary and peritoneal TB; in a recent report, 21 of 211 patients with peritoneal TB died during follow-up.[39]

Awareness and knowledge about the disease, high index of suspicion and appropriate management can reduce the mortality of TB, including abdominal TB.

> **Key Point**
>
> 1. Clinical features of abdominal TB include general symptoms of the disease, and abdominal pain, distension, bowel disturbance, and the presence of a palpable mass or ascites.

REFERENCES

1. Shah SR, Shenai S, Desai DC, et al. Comparison of *Mycobacterium tuberculosis* culture using liquid culture medium and Lowenstein Jensen medium in abdominal tuberculosis. Indian J Gastroenterol. 2010;29(6):237-9.
2. Tripathi PB, Amarapurkar AD. Morphological spectrum of gastrointestinal tuberculosis. Trop Gastroenterol. 2009;30(1):35-9.
3. Gadodia A, Sharma R, Jeyaseelan N. Tuberculous abdominal cocoon. Am J Trop Med Hyg. 2011;84(1):1-2.
4. Bhalla AS, Hari S, Chandrashekhara SH, et al. Abdominal lymphatic tuberculosis and portal hypertension. Gastroenterol Clin Biol. 2010;34(12):696-701.
5. Tan KK, Chen K, Liau KH, et al. Pancreatic tuberculosis mimicking pancreatic carcinoma: series of three cases. Eur J Gastroenterol Hepatol. 2009;21(11):1317-9.
6. Singh B, Saxena PD, Kumar V, et al. Tubercular liver abscess in immuno-competent patients. J Assoc Physicians India. 2011;59:523-4.
7. Dixit R, Arya MK, Panjabi M, et al. Clinical profile of patients having splenic involvement in tuberculosis. Indian J Tuberc. 2010;57(1):25-30.
8. Govindasamy M, Srinivasan T, Varma V, et al. Biliary tract tuberculosis—a diagnostic dilemma. J Gastrointest Surg. 2011;15(12):2172-7.
9. Kapoor VK, Gupta S, Sikora SS, et al. Acute tubercular abdomen. Indian J Surg. 1991;53:71-5.
10. Bhansali SK. Abdominal tuberculosis. Experiences with 300 cases. Am J Gastroenterol. 1977;67(4):324-37.
11. Adhikari S, Hossein MZ, Das A, et al. Etiology and outcome of acute intestinal obstruction: a review of 367 patients in Eastern India. Saudi J Gastroenterol. 2010;16(4):285-7.
12. Sharma LK, Gupta S, Soin AS, et al. Generalised peritonitis—the tropical spectrum. Japanese Journal of Surgery. 1991;21:272-7.
13. Kapoor VK, Kriplani AK, Chattopadhyay TK, et al. Tuberculous perforations of the small intestine. Indian J Tubercul. 1986;33:188-9.
14. Sinhasan SP, Puranik RB, Kulkarni MH. Abdominal tuberculosis may masquerade many diseases. Saudi J Gastroenterol. 2011;17(2):110-3.

15. Shao H, Yang ZG, Deng W, et al. Tuberculosis versus lymphoma in the abdominal lymph nodes: a comparative study using contrast-enhanced MRI. Eur J Radiol. 2012;81(10):2513-7.

16. Wu CH, Changchien CC, Tseng CW, et al. Disseminated peritoneal tuberculosis simulating advanced ovarian cancer: a retrospective study of 17 cases. Taiwan J Obstet Gynecol. 2011;50(3):292-6.

17. Kaya M, Kaplan MA, Isikdogan A, et al. Differentiation of tuberculous peritonitis from peritonitis carcinomatosa without surgical intervention. Saudi J Gastroenterol. 2011;17(5):312-7.

18. Shah P, Ramakantan R. Role of vasculitis in the natural history of abdominal tuberculosis—evaluation by mesenteric angiography. Indian J Gastroenterol. 1991;10:127-30.

19. Yachha SK, Misra S, Malik AK, et al. Spectrum of malabsorption syndrome in north Indian children. Indian J Gastroenetrol. 1993;12:120-5.

20. Kapoor VK, Chattopadhyay TK, Sharma LK. Radiology of abdominal tuberculosis. Australas Radiol. 1988;32(3):365-7.

21. Zhang M, Li M, Xu GP, et al. Neoplasm-like abdominal nonhematogenous disseminated tuberculous lymphadenopathy: CT evaluation of 12 cases and literature review. World J Gastroenterol. 2011;17(35):4038-43.

22. Chen CJ, Yao WJ, Chou CY, et al. Peritoneal tuberculosis with elevated serum CA125 mimicking peritoneal carcinomatosis on F-18 FDG-PET/CT. Ann Nucl Med. 2008;22(6):525-7.

23. Tian G, Xiao Y, Chen B, et al. Multi-site abdominal tuberculosis mimics malignancy on ^{18}F-FDG PET/CT: report of three cases. World J Gastroenterol. 2010;16(33):4237-42.

24. Dhir V, Mathew P, Bhandari S, et al. Endosonography-guided fine needle aspiration cytology of intra-abdominal lymph nodes with unknown primary in a tuberculosis endemic region. J Gastroenterol Hepatol. 2011;26(12):1721-4.

25. Puri R, Mangla R, Eloubeidi M, et al. Diagnostic yield of EUS-guided FNA and cytology in suspected tubercular intra-abdominal lymphadenopathy. Gastrointest Endosc. 2012;75(5):1005-10.

26. Mehta PK, Raj A, Singh N, et al. Diagnosis of extrapulmonary tuberculosis by PCR. FEMS Immunol Med Microbiol. 2012;66(1):20-36.

27. Bhargava DK, Gupta M, Nijhawan S, et al. Adenosine deaminase (ADA) in peritoneal tuberculosis: diagnostic value in ascitic fluid and serum. Tubercle. 1990;71(2):121-6.

28. Dwivedi M, Misra SP, Misra V, et al. Value of adenosine deaminase estimation in the diagnosis of tuberculous ascites. Am J Gastroenterol. 1990;85:1123-5.

29. Khan FY, Al-Muzrakchi AM, Elbedawi MM, et al. Peritoneal tuberculosis in Qatar: a five-year hospital-based study from 2005 to 2009. Travel Med Infect Dis. 2012;10(1):25-31.

30. Malik AM, Talpur KA, Soomro AG, et al. Yield of diagnostic laparoscopy in abdominal tuberculosis: is it worth attempting? Surg Laparosc Endosc Percutan Tech. 2011;21(3):191-3.

31. Mandal A, Das SK, Bairagya TD. Presenting experience of managing abdominal tuberculosis at a tertiary care hospital in India. J Glob Infect Dis. 2011;3(4):344-7.

32. Horne NW. Problems of tuberculosis in decline. Br Med J (Clin Res Ed). 1984;288(6426):1249-51.

33. Vyas K, Rathi P. Human immunodeficiency virus and abdominal tuberculosis—dual partners in a crime. J Assoc Physicians India. 1999;47(3):309-12.

34. Rathi PM, Amarapurakar DN, Parikh SS, et al. Impact of human immunodeficiency virus infection on abdominal tuberculosis in western India. J Clin Gastroenterol. 1997;24(1):43-8.
35. Balasubramanian R, Nagarajan M, Balambal R, et al. Randomised controlled clinical trial of short course chemotherapy in abdominal tuberculosis: a five-year report. Int J Tuberc Lung Dis. 1997;1(1):44-51.
36. Katariya RN, Sood S, Rao PG, et al. Strictureplasty for tubercular strictures of the gastrointestinal tract. Br J Surg. 1977;64:496-8.
37. Sircar S, Taneja VA, Kansra U. Epidemiology and clinical presentation of abdominal tuberculosis—a retrospective study. J Indian Med Assoc. 1996;94(9):342-4.
38. Chen HL, Wu MS, Chang WH, et al. Abdominal tuberculosis in south-eastern Taiwan: 20 years of experience. J Formos Med Assoc. 2009;108(3):195-201.
39. Yeh HF, Chiu TF, Chen JC, et al. Tuberculous peritonitis: analysis of 211 cases in Taiwan. Dig Liver Dis. 2012;44(2):111-7.

SUGGESTED READINGS

1. Kapoor VK. Abdominal tuberculosis. Postgraduate Medical Journal. 1998;74:459-67.
2. Kapoor VK. Koch's or Crohn's. Int (Br) J Clin Pract. 1997;51:246-7.
3. Kapoor VK, Sharma LK. Abdominal tuberculosis. Br J Surg. 1988;75:2-3.
4. Sharma MP, Bhatia V. Abdominal tuberculosis. Indian J Med Res. 2004;120:305-15.
5. Tandon HD, Prakash A. Pathology of intestinal tuberculosis and its distinction from Crohn's disease. Gut. 1972;13:260-9.

13

Management of the Diabetic Foot

K Mylankal, CP Shearman

INTRODUCTION

Diabetes mellitus (DM) is a chronic disorder of glucose metabolism with multisystem involvement and serious long-term consequences. The prevalence of diabetes shows geographical variations, being low prevalence in rural developing nations, intermediate in developed nations and high in certain ethnic groups. However, globally there is a notable increase in the incidence of DM and this trend is closely linked to population growth, urbanisation, obesity and physical inactivity. By 2030, it is estimated that the number of diabetic people worldwide will increase from 336 million currently to 552 million (8.3% of adult population).[1] In England alone, there are over 3 million people diagnosed with diabetes which accounts for 5.5% of the adult population with a further 2% remaining undiagnosed.[2] It is estimated that currently 11% of the total health care budget which equates to £2.3−2.5 billion is spent on diabetic care and these figures will have to increase to keep up with the future demands.

Diabetes accelerates and modifies the atherosclerotic process and is a major risk factor for the development of atherosclerotic peripheral arterial disease (PAD). Diabetic patients are 4 times more likely to develop PAD and 8% of patients with type 2 DM already have PAD at the time of initial diagnosis.[3,4] A patient with PAD and DM has a 70−80% increased risk of dying from cardiovascular disease compared to a person with diabetes and no PAD. In addition, the risk of lower limb amputation is 10−16 times greater in people with diabetes.[5]

EPIDEMIOLOGY

Foot sepsis is a common complication leading to hospitalisation of a diabetic patient and this often culminates in amputation. Globally, over a million people lose a leg to diabetes related complications every year; in simple terms this equates to one lower limb every 30 seconds and this figure is increasing.[6] In addition, diabetic complications of foot ulceration and sepsis account for significant morbidity and between 15% and 25% of all diabetics will suffer foot ulceration during their lifetime.[7] These ulcers take from weeks to months to heal and some cases may never heal at all. In addition, upto 80% of diabetic individuals with previous foot ulceration are likely to have recurrent ulceration over the next 5 years.[8,9] Diabetic foot complications requiring in-patient hospitalisation, antimicrobial therapy, topical dressings, orthotic footwear and time away from work have significant cost implications to the community and individual. With the increasing prevalence of diabetes, the vascular surgeon will encounter a larger case load of patients with diabetes related PAD and foot complications in the future. It is hence imperative that we are well equipped to deal promptly and effectively with this patient cohort to reduce morbidity and mortality. In this chapter, authors have examined the modern trends in the management of the diabetic foot and identified key areas that need focus to improve the overall outcome.

> **Key Point**
>
> Incidence of diabetes is increasing worldwide.

PATHOGENESIS

Diabetic foot complications are a result of ischaemia, neuropathy and infection. The pattern of PAD in DM is different to the non-diabetic patient.[10] There is predominantly small vessel involvement below the knee with relative sparing of the proximal aorto-iliac segments[11] and the foot vessels. Neuropathy affects the pain and temperature fibres initially and exposes the insensate foot to minor trauma. The motor innervations to the intrinsic foot muscles are affected and the overriding effect of the long flexors of the foot produces clawing with exaggerated pressure points over the plantar aspect of the metatarsophalangeal joints. Neuropathy of the autonomic outflow causes dysfunction of skin sweat glands and sebaceous glands. The dry cracked skin can then be a portal for entry of pathogens. In addition, involvement of the proprioceptive nerve fibres contributes to joint deformity of the foot and ankle joints which often coexists with diabetic foot ulcers.[12] Thickening of the capillary basement membrane is seen in DM and this obtunds neutrophil migration and the response of the tissue to infection.[13] In addition, abnormal vasomotor control with loss of axon reflex and impaired vasodilation after injury has a cumulative effect in dampening tissue response to infection.

CLINICAL PRESENTATION AND EXAMINATION

The diabetic patient with PAD can present with symptoms of intermittent claudication or rest pain. Although the patient may have these symptoms of vascular insufficiency, more often they present with foot ulceration or infections. A meticulous examination of the foot should include examination for skin changes of cyanosis, erythema and dependent rubor, skin and nail atrophy, hair loss, peripheral oedema and temperature gradient. Examination

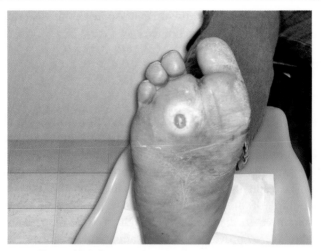

Figure 13.1: Typical neuropathic ulcer on sole of foot

of foot pulses and capillary refill time in addition to a simple bedside test of ankle brachial pressure index is mandatory.

The neuropathic foot has the characteristic appearance of dry cracked skin with calluses on the pressure points and clawing of the toes (Fig. 13.1). The foot may appear warm and hyperaemic despite significant ischaemia in cases where there is abnormal arteriovenous shunting due to autonomic dysfunction. In some instances, patients present with a painful neuropathic foot which is a manifestation of the deranged glucose metabolism. Neuropathic assessment using a 10-gram monofilament is highly predictive of the foot at risk of ulceration.[7,14] In addition, the tuning fork (128 Hz) test may help identify patients with diminished vibration perception although this test may not be so beneficial.

Diabetic patients presenting with ulcers need a thorough examination of the foot to determine ulcer extent, position in relation to bony prominences, and the presence of infection, ischaemia and neuropathy. A systematic classification of ulcers helps in comparing data and although there are many classification systems, most are based around extent of ulcer, perfusion and infection. Foot sepsis may be associated with local signs and symptoms of inflammation although sometimes this may be obtunded by poor leucocyte function, PAD and neuropathy. Often, worsening glycaemic control may be an indicator of an infective process in the foot. A swollen red foot with chronic ulceration indicates an ongoing infective process. However, sepsis may track along the deeper plantar planes of the foot with minimal involvement of the dorsum. Careful foot examination for tenderness, fluctuant areas and surgical emphysema may reveal deep seated collections. Inflammatory blood markers such as white blood cell count, erythrocyte sedimentation rate and C-reactive protein are elevated in only half of diabetic patients with deep seated infections.[15,16] Osteomyelitis should be suspected when an ulcer overlying a bony prominence fails to heal despite optimal therapy or when the toes become deformed and indurated.

DIAGNOSTIC INVESTIGATIONS

Vascular Investigations

Ankle brachial pressure index (ABPI) is a useful non-invasive bedside test that often helps to identify the critically ischaemic limb. Severe ischemia has an ABPI less than 0.4–0.45 with an absolute ankle systolic pressure less than 55 mmHg. However, non-compressible vessels from diabetic arteriosclerosis result in spuriously high values and this may be the case in upto one-third of diabetic patients.[17] Toe pressure measurements are a useful alternative in these cases although in 16% of patients; this was not achievable due to previous toe amputations, ulcerations or pain.[17] Toe pressure less than 30 mmHg indicates that revascularisation is essential to promote tissue healing.[18] Transcutaneous oxygen pressure (TcPO$_2$) may be a useful adjunct to help the decision-making process for revascularisation although local factors such as peripheral oedema can make interpretation inaccurate. Tissue healing is likely to occur on conservative measures with a TcPO$_2$ greater than 50 mmHg and revascularisation is warranted for a TcPO$_2$ less than 30 mmHg.

Extensive calcification of the arterial wall associated with diabetic arteriosclerosis poses challenges in interpretation of arterial duplex and CT angiogram images (Fig. 13.2). Magnetic resonance imaging (MRI) with

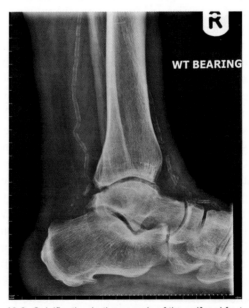

Figure 13.2: Calcification in the vessels of the calf and foot arteries

gadolinium contrast has its limitations in the diabetic patient with renal impairment due to the risk of nephrogenic systemic fibrosis but is emerging as the optimum method of vessel imaging. Intra-arterial digital subtraction angiography is still frequently required. Selective cannulation of the relevant supply vessel helps acquire excellent images of the distal foot vessels and is often essential for preoperative planning. Iso-osmolar contrast is widely used to limit the nephrotoxic insult in the diabetic individual. Metformin can induce lactic acidosis and hence should be withheld prior to contrast angiography.[19] In addition, adequate prehydration and alkalinisation with sodium bicarbonate infusion are recommended to protect against the effects of contrast induced nephrotoxicity.[20] However, the role of N-acetylcysteine in averting nephrotoxicity following contrast use is unproven.

Soft Tissue Infection and Osteomyelitis

Imaging studies are vital to identify underlying infection. Plain radiographs may show foreign bodies, gas shadows or bone involvement (Fig. 13.3). Periosteal elevation, loss of cortical bone with erosions, new bone formation and bone sclerosis are all indicative of osteomyelitis in the diabetic foot. However, the sensitivity of plain radiograph in predicting osteomyelitis varies between 25% and 75%. Overall, radiographic changes are marginally predictive of osteomyelitis when positive or less so when negative and changes noted from serial radiographs over a period of time are a better predictor of osteomyelitis.[21] Magnetic resonance imaging has a 77 – 100% sensitivity for detection of osteomyelitis and deep-seated foot infection although a lower specificity due to its inability to differentiate it from fractures.[22] Low

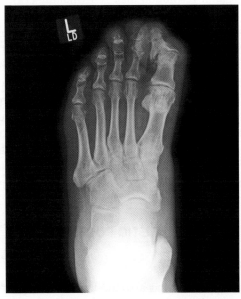

Figure 13.3: Bone destruction indicating osteomyelitis

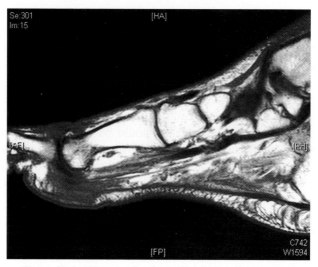

Figure 13.4: MR scan of patient with infection in metatarsal

intensity focal signals on T1-weighted images, high focal signals on T2-weighted images and high bone marrow signals are some of the features highly suggestive of osteomyelitis on MRI (Fig. 13.4). Radiolabelled white cell scans have a high sensitivity and specificity for osteomyelitis.[23,24] Normal bone does not absorb radiolabelled white cells and high concentration of white cells in the bone is indicative of an infective process. Hence, labelled white cell scanning gives superior results to bone scan in the diagnosis of osteomyelitis. White cell labelling with ^{99m}Tc (Technefium-99m)appears to produce better spatial resolution than ^{111}I (Indium-111), and the sensitivity and specificity almost matches that of MRI.

Bone biopsy is the most reliable method to diagnose bone infection (Technetium-99m) and in addition, it helps to identify the pathogenic organism and also gives information on antibiotic sensitivity profile.[25] A recent retrospective multicentre study comparing antibiotic use based on sensitivity profile from bone samples versus soft tissue showed a significantly better clinical outcome from the bone biopsy group.[26] However, bone biopsy can be prone to misleading results due to sampling errors or recent antibiotic use. The role of bone biopsy is diminishing although there are instances when it is helpful especially when there is uncertainty in the diagnosis, or failure of current antibiotic therapy where the sensitivity profile will help to choose the appropriate antibiotic.

TREATMENT OF THE DIABETIC FOOT

Medical Management

A multimodality approach and a sound understanding of the aetiology are essential to obtain favourable outcomes in the diabetic foot. Aggressive glycaemia control may often warrant switching to insulin, and this may be preferable inpatients with active infections, those awaiting radiological contrast studies and surgery. Primary prevention strategies need to address other risk factors such as anti-platelet therapy, smoking, hypercholesterolemia and hypertension. In addition, patient directed educational strategies help in the long-term care of the patient with diabetes and a foot complication.

The mainstay of treatment in neuropathic ulcer is restricted weight bearing. In the uncomplicated ulcer this may be accomplished in an outpatient setting with topical dressing care, and weight offloading which can be achieved by using protective footwear, insoles, orthosis, total contact cast, walkers, crutches and wheelchair. However, non-compliance and infective complications may necessitate inpatient admission for aggressive antibiotic therapy, strict bed rest and management of ischaemia.

Infection Control

Infected ulcers are an indication for antibiotic therapy although antibiotics are not always required for the chronic ulcer with polymicrobial colonisation. An empiric broad-spectrum antibiotic cover is initiated based on local preferences which can subsequently be changed to target a specific pathogen.

Limb threatening infection in the diabetic patient is an emergency which requires hospital admission, bed rest and debridement. Empiric antibiotic therapy is commenced which is tailored based on sensitivities from deeper tissue samples. Superficial wound swabs are notoriously unreliable. Although trials have looked at the efficacy of various antibiotic regimens, in the context of hospital acquired MRSA infections, vancomycin is the ideal choice for empirical treatment.[27] In addition, fluoroquinolones which cover gram-negative and gram-positive pathogens and metronidazole with its anaerobic activity are recommended as a combination.[28] Moderate to severe infections may often require a longer duration of therapy for 3 weeks.[29] Antibiotic therapy for osteomyelitis is often for a protracted course of weeks to years in some cases although the recurrence rates are very high.

Severe foot infection with purulent malodorous discharge, crepitus and extensive gangrene are suggestive of necrotising fasciitis which requires emergency surgery. The confined spaces in the foot result in rapidly ascending infection which can lead to systemic sepsis, and hence any delay in surgical debridement should be avoided. Debridement is aimed at removing non-viable infected tissue and reduces the septic load. Tendon sheaths are milked to drain any collection and excised if involved. Liberal incisions are made to ensure adequate drainage.

Key Point

Severe diabetic foot infection requires emergency surgical attention.

There are a number of topical wound care modalities currently available to help healing of chronic wounds. Hyperbaric oxygen therapy has been used for sometime. It is expensive and not all patients are suitable for it, but there is some evidence that hyperbaric oxygen therapy offers significantly higher wound healing and limb salvage rate in diabetic foot ulcer patients.[30,31] Topical negative pressure wound therapy has been widely investigated and trials have shown clear benefits in healing rate and healing time.[32,33] However, there has been very variable uptake of these technologies and recent NICE guidelines and a Cochrane review have concluded that there is currently insufficient data to support the cost-effectiveness of these treatments in everyday use and further clinical trials are needed to identify their role.

Revascularisation Options

The diabetic patient with PAD poses specific challenges related to the anatomical distribution of atherosclerosis which predominantly affects vessels below the knee. Inflow for the distal bypass can be from superficial femoral artery or the popliteal artery as the proximal vasculature is often spared in diabetic PAD. However distally, the below knee run-off vessels are diseased and should be carefully chosen to ensure uninterrupted flow into the foot and preferably the artery supplying the anatomical region of the ulcer. Calcification can often make the distal anastomosis challenging and if the vessel wall is hard and calcified but not occluded it can, with care, be used as a recipient vessel for bypass graft. Vessel lumen occluders may be less traumatic than the use of clamps on the calcified vessel at the time of the procedure. Autologous veins provide the best long-term results with secondary patency rates of the saphenous vein graft being superior to other conduits. The most comprehensive study of distal bypasses with greater than 1,000 pedal revascularisation procedures had primary patency, secondary patency and limb salvage rates of 56.8%, 62.7% and 78.2% at 5 years.[34] Although surgical bypass is still commonly used for distal revascularisation, advances in endovascular techniques have improved the results of below knee interventions. Because of the morbidity associated with open surgery in an increasingly older patient group with other cardiovascular co-morbidities, the endovascular approach becomes more attractive. This becomes all the more relevant as only 14–22% of patients have a patent graft, healed ulcer and remain fully ambulant at 42 months following a distal bypass.[35] The bypass versus angioplasty in severe ischaemia of the leg (BASIL) trial which randomised 452 with limb ischaemia included 42% patients with diabetes.[36] Amputation-free survival and mortality were similar in both groups in the medium term although the recommendation was to offer

Key Points

- Distal revascularisation is critical for ischaemic ulcer healing.
- Endovascular and distal bypass options are complementary to each other.

endovascular treatment for patients with significant comorbidities and life expectancy less than 2 years. The longer term results favour surgery, with angioplasty requiring repeat interventions. Two meta-analyses of angioplasty compared to crural bypass in a predominantly diabetic cohort have reported similar limb salvage rate after both interventions although primary and secondary intervention rates were higher in the angioplasty group.[37,38]

The choice between the two revascularisation procedure (distal bypass and endovascular interventions) is often based on patient co-morbidities, fitness to undergo prolonged surgical procedure, complexity of the arterial disease and local experience. The BASIL trial showed that only 29% of patients are suitable for both endovascular and bypass procedures, and hence these two complement each other. The best modality of revascularisation is often decided by the needs of each individual patient.

Amputation Versus Limb Salvage

Amputation is aimed at removing infected or gangrenous tissue and helps create a functional foot or stump for weight bearing. Toe or transmetatarsal amputations usually provide a functional foot for walking. Extensive tissue loss with failure of wound healing even after revascularisation is an indication for major amputation. Preservation of stump length is critical for future ambulation and a below knee stump is preferred whenever possible. An above knee amputation is indicated in patients with dementia, bed bound with fixed contractures of the knee and hip joint and a short life expectancy.

The decision between amputation and limb salvage is often determined by factors such as patient expectation and co-morbidities. The younger patient with high expectations may be able to live a near normal life with an amputation unlike the diabetic patient with associated cardiac and peripheral vascular disease whose expectations are to remain independent with limb salvage and not be wheelchair bound.[39] An individual's pre-amputation mobility is a key determinant to performance following an amputation. They are less likely to use prosthesis if they were house bound previously, older than 60 or had coronary artery disease.[40] The algorithm for both limb salvage and amputation rely on ensuring adequate blood supply, infection control and providing biomechanical stability.

> **Key Point**
>
> Multidisciplinary team approach improves outcome in the diabetic foot.

Multidisciplinary Team Approach

The complexity of DM with multiorgan involvement warrants a multidisciplinary approach to the management of the diabetic foot. This team comprises of specialists with relevant skills who work together and include a medical diabetologist, vascular and orthopaedic surgeons, podiatrists, diabetic specialist nurse and orthotists. A protocol driven multidisciplinary approach with emphasis on patient education reduces the incidence of diabetic foot complications. Comparative cohort studies have shown a significant reduction in amputation rates following introduction of multidisciplinary team review, and upto 85% of amputations are preventable by this approach.[14]

Key Points

1. Incidence of diabetes is increasing worldwide.

2. Severe diabetic foot infection requires emergency surgical attention.

3. Distal revascularisation is critical for ischaemic ulcer healing.

4. Endovascular and distal bypass options are complementary to each other.

5. Multidisciplinary team approach improves outcome in the diabetic foot.

REFERENCES

1. Shaw JE, Sicree RA, Zimmet PZ. Global estimates of the prevalence of diabetes for 2010 and 2030. Diabetes Res Clin Pract. 2009;87(1):4-14.

2. Kerr M. (2011). Inpatient care for people with diabetes. The economic case for change. [online] Available from www.nhs.diabetes.uk.

3. Newman AB, Siscovick DS, Manolio TA, et al. Ankle-arm index as a marker of atherosclerosis in the cardiovascular health study. Cardiovascular Heart Study (CHS) Collaborative Research Group. Circulation. 1993;88(3):837-45.

4. Gregg EW, Sorlie P, Paulose-Ram R, et al. Prevalence of lower-extremity disease in the US adult population ≥40 years of age with and without diabetes: 1999-2000 national health and nutrition examination survey. Diabetes Care. 2004;27(7):1591-7.

5. Al-Delaimy WK, Merchant AT, Rimm EB, et al. Effect of type 2 diabetes and its duration on the risk of peripheral arterial disease among men. Am J Med. 2004;116(4):236-40.

6. Boulton AJ, Vileikyte L, Ragnarson-Tennvall G, et al. The global burden of diabetic foot disease. Lancet. 2005;366(9498):1719-24.

7. Singh N, Armstrong DG, Lipsky BA. Preventing foot ulcers in patients with diabetes. JAMA. 2005;293(2):217-28.

8. Peters EJ, Armstrong DG, Lavery LA. Risk factors for recurrent diabetic foot ulcers: site matters. Diabetes Care. 2007;30(8):2077-9.

9. Chantelau E, Kushner T, Spraul M. How effective is cushioned therapeutic footwear in protecting diabetic feet? A clinical study. Diabet Med. 1990;7(4):355-9.

10. Amos AF, McCarty DJ, Zimmet P. The rising global burden of diabetes and its complications: estimates and projections to the year 2010. Diabet Med. 1997;14(Suppl 5):S1-85.

11. Mueller T, Haidinger D, Luft C, et al. Association between erythrocyte mean corpuscular volume and peripheral arterial disease in male subjects: a case control study. Angiology. 2001;52(9):605-13.

12. Schon LC, Easley ME, Weinfeld SB. Charcot neuroarthropathy of the foot and ankle. Clin Orthop Relat Res. 1998;349:116-31.

13. Rayman G, Williams SA, Spencer PD, et al. Impaired microvascular hyperaemic response to minor skin trauma in type I diabetes. Br Med J (Clin Res Ed). 1986;292(6531):1295-8.

14. Apelqvist J, Bakker K, van Houtum WH, et al. Practical guidelines on the management and prevention of the diabetic foot: based upon the International Consensus on the Diabetic Foot (2007) prepared by the International Working

Group on the Diabetic Foot. Diabetes Metab Res Rev. 2008;24(Suppl 1):S181-7.

15. Eneroth M, Larsson J, Apelqvist J. Deep foot infections in patients with diabetes and foot ulcer: an entity with different characteristics, treatments, and prognosis. J Diabetes Complications. 1999;13(5-6):254-63.

16. Lipsky BA, Berendt AR, Embil J, et al. Diagnosing and treating diabetic foot infections. Diabetes Metab Res Rev. 2004;20(Suppl 1):S56-64.

17. Faqlia E, Clerici G, Clerissi J, et al. Long-term prognosis of diabetic patients with critical limb ischemia: a population-based cohort study. Diabetes Care. 2009;32(5):822-7.

18. Takolander R, Rauwerda JA. The use of non-invasive vascular assessment in diabetic patients with foot lesions. Diabet Med. 1996;13(Suppl 1):S39-42.

19. Heikkinen M, Salmenperä M, Lepäntalo A, et al. Diabetes care for patients with peripheral arterial disease. Eur J Vasc Endovasc Surg. 2007;33(5):583-91.

20. Pomposelli F. Arterial imaging in patients with lower-extremity ischemia and diabetes mellitus. J Am Podiatr Med Assoc. 2010;100(5):412-23.

21. Butalia S, Palda VA, Sargeant RJ, et al., Does this patient with diabetes have osteomyelitis of the lower extremity? JAMA. 2008;299(7):806-13.

22. Kapoor A, Page S, Lavalley M, et al. Magnetic resonance imaging for diagnosing foot osteomyelitis: a meta-analysis. Arch Intern Med. 2007;167(2):125-32.

23. Palestro CJ, Love C. Nuclear medicine and diabetic foot infections. Semin Nucl Med. 2009;39(1):52-65.

24. Capriotti G, Chianelli M, Signore A. Nuclear medicine imaging of diabetic foot infection: results of meta-analysis. Nucl Med Commun. 2006;27(10):757-64.

25. Peters EJ, Lipsky BA, Berendt AR, et al. A systematic review of the effectiveness of interventions in the management of infection in the diabetic foot. Diabetes Metab Res Rev. 2012;28(Suppl 1):142-62.

26. Senneville E, Lombart A, Beltrand E, et al. Outcome of diabetic foot osteomyelitis treated nonsurgically: a retrospective cohort study. Diabetes Care. 2008;31(4):637-42.

27. Lipsky BA. Empirical therapy for diabetic foot infections: are there clinical clues to guide antibiotic selection? Clin Microbiol Infect. 2007;13(4):351-3.

28. Ellison MJ. Vancomycin, metronidazole, and tetracyclines. Clin Podiatr Med Surg. 1992;9(2):425-42.

29. Lipsky BA, Berendt AR, Deery HG, et al. Diagnosis and treatment of diabetic foot infections. Clin Infect Dis. 2004;39(7):885-910.

30. Kessler L, Bilbault P, Ortéga F, et al. Hyperbaric oxygenation accelerates the healing rate of nonischemic chronic diabetic foot ulcers: a prospective randomized study. Diabetes Care. 2003;26(8):2378-82.

31. Duzgun AP, Satir HZ, Ozozan O, et al. Effect of hyperbaric oxygen therapy on healing of diabetic foot ulcers. J Foot Ankle Surg. 2008;47(6):515-9.

32. Armstrong DG, Lavery LA. Negative pressure wound therapy after partial diabetic foot amputation: a multicentre, randomised controlled trial. Lancet. 2005;366(9498):1704-10.

33. Apelqvist J, Armstrong DG, Lavery LA, et al. Resource utilization and economic costs of care based on a randomized trial of vacuum-assisted closure therapy in the treatment of diabetic foot wounds. Am J Surg. 2008;195(6):782-8.

34. Pomposelli FB, Kansal N, Hamdan AD, et al. A decade of experience with dorsalis pedis artery bypass: analysis of outcome in more than 1000 cases. J Vasc Surg. 2003;37(2):307-15.

35. Nicoloff AD, Taylor LM Jr, McLafferty RB, et al. Patient recovery after infrainguinal bypass grafting for limb salvage. J Vasc Surg. 1998;27(2):256-63; discussion 264-6.

36. Adam DJ, Beard JD, Cleveland T, et al. Bypass versus angioplasty in severe ischaemia of the leg (BASIL): multicentre, randomised controlled trial. Lancet. 2005;366(9501):1925-34.

37. Romiti M, Albers M, Brochado-Neto FC, et al. Meta-analysis of infrapopliteal angioplasty for chronic critical limb ischemia. J Vasc Surg. 2008;47(5):975-81.

38. Albers M, Romiti M, Brochado-Neto FC, et al. Meta-analysis of popliteal-to-distal vein bypass grafts for critical ischemia. J Vasc Surg. 2006;43(3):498-503.

39. Buzato MA, Tribulatto EC, Costa SM, et al. Major amputations of the lower leg. The patients two years later. Acta Chir Belg. 2002;102(4):248-52.

40. Taylor SM, Kalbaugh CA, Blackhurst DW, et al. Preoperative clinical factors predict postoperative functional outcomes after major lower limb amputation: an analysis of 553 consecutive patients. J Vasc Surg. 2005;42(2):227-35.

14 | Randomised Clinical Trials and Meta-analyses in Surgery

Siân Pugh

This chapter summarises the selection of randomised clinical trials (RCTs) and meta-analyses relevant to surgery published in 2011.

GENERAL

Appendicitis

Interest has grown in the use of antibiotics as the first-line management of acute appendicitis. A non-inferiority RCT was undertaken in 243 patients aged 18–68 years with acute uncomplicated appendicitis as diagnosed by CT scan.[1] Incidence of 30-day postintervention peritonitis was significantly more frequent in the antibiotic group (8%, n = 9) than in the appendicectomy group (2%, n = 2; treatment difference 5.8; 95% CI 0.3–12.1). As such antibiotic treatment with amoxicillin plus clavulanic acid was inferior to emergency appendicectomy for the treatment of acute uncomplicated appendicitis.

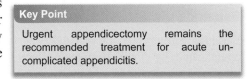

Key Point

Urgent appendicectomy remains the recommended treatment for acute uncomplicated appendicitis.

Hernias

The incidence of postoperative pain is a consideration when selecting the type and method of fixation of mesh for hernia repair. An RCT reported that mesh fixation with fibrin sealant in laparoscopic ventral hernia repair results in less postoperative pain and a shorter convalescence than tack fixation.[2] However, no long-term follow-up is available. Another trial randomised patients to either absorbable polyglycolic acid 3/0 sutures (Dexon®) or 1 mL butyl-2-cyanoacrylate tissue glue for fixation of a lightweight (LW) mesh during local anaesthetic Lichtenstein hernia repair.[3] The use of tissue glue did not reduce postoperative pain.

Two trials have compared types of mesh. In a four-arm RCT, pure middleweight (MW) polypropylene mesh, an LW composite polypropylene mesh, or a titanised lightweight (TLW) mesh were compared with a standard heavyweight (HW) mesh.[4] One year after transabdominal preperitoneal

(TAPP) repair, frequency of pain did not differ between the groups. By contrast, a different trial found that LW nonwoven polypropylene mesh, when compared with a HW polypropylene mesh, resulted in reduced postoperative pain in the short-term (upto 3 months) after Lichtenstein inguinal hernioplasty.[5] No difference in recurrence rate was observed at 12- and 60-month follow-up.

Finally, a trial compared the Lichtenstein and laparoscopic TAPP repair of recurrent inguinal hernias.[6] Comparisons were made for several preoperative, intraoperative and postoperative factors; however, none of the results reached significance. This may be due to the small numbers involved in the trial, just 52 patients in total.

Wound Closure

Incisional hernia remains a frequent cause of morbidity following abdominal wound closure. One study hypothesised that a nonabsorbable suture (Prolene[®]) would result in fewer incisional hernias than a slowly absorbed suture (PDS[®]) following closure of a midline laparotomy wound, whilst not causing other complications such as suture sinus or surgical site infection.[7] At a median follow-up of 31 months, the incidence of incisional hernia was 20.2% (45/223) for Prolene[®] and 24.9% (58/223) with PDS[®] (p = 0.229). Whilst the incidence of incisional hernia was higher than expected the hypothesis was not proven.

OESOPHAGOGASTRIC

Bariatric

Bariatric surgery is increasingly performed in patients with obesity complicated by Type II diabetes mellitus (T2DM). A trial studied the surgical treatment of 60 non-morbidly obese patients [body mas index (BMI) < 35] with poorly controlled T2DM comparing gastric bypass with sleeve gastrectomy.[8] The primary outcome of remission of T2DM was achieved by 28 (93%) in the gastric bypass group and 14 (47%) in the sleeve gastrectomy group (p = 0.02). Of note patients with BMI 25–35 would not meet current National Institute of Clinical Excellence (NICE) criteria for bariatric surgery.[9]

> **Key Point**
>
> In patients with BMI 25–35, gastric bypass is more likely to achieve remission of T2DM than sleeve gastrectomy.

Gastro-Oesophageal Reflux Disease

Division of the short gastric vessels during Nissen 360° fundoplication may be relevant to the development of certain postoperative complications.[10,11] A meta-analysis included five trials of division versus no division of the short gastric vessels comprising a total of 388 operations.[12] There was no difference in the outcome measures of reoperation, length of hospital stay, postoperative dysphagia, reflux and gas bloat syndrome. A second meta-analysis included just the two largest RCTs and focused on the long-term symptomatic outcomes.[13] At 10–12 years follow-up, there were no differences in symptoms of heartburn or dysphagia, ability to belch or vomit, and use of anti-secretory medications. However, division was associated with a higher rate of bloating symptoms (72% vs 48%; p = 0.002). Whilst these data challenge the belief that division of the short gastric vessels is an essential part of the procedure, an adequately powered prospective trial is needed.

Oesophagogastric Malignancy

Adenocarcinoma

Barrett's oesophagus is a risk factor for the development of oesophageal adenocarcinoma. High-grade dysplasia (HGD) and early cancer (EC) limited to the mucosa in Barrett's can be effectively treated by endoscopic resection, avoiding the need for oesophagectomy. In order to reduce the incidence of metachronous lesions, complete eradication of the metaplastic epithelium is recommended using either stepwise radical endoscopic resection (SRER) or radiofrequency ablation (RFA).[14-19] A total of 49 patients with short segment Barrett's (≤ 5 cm) containing HGD/EC were randomised to SRER or ER/RFA.[20] Both yielded equivalent rates of complete histological response for neoplasia (100% SRER and 96% ER/RFA) and complete histological response for intestinal metaplasia (92% SRER and 96% ER/RFA). However, SRER was associated with a significantly higher stenosis rate (SRER 88% vs ER/RFA 14%; p < 0.001); therefore, ER/RFA may be the preferred method.

Squamous Cell Carcinoma

The majority of patients undergoing surgical resection of oesophageal squamous cell carcinoma (SCC) receive neoadjuvant treatment [chemotherapy or chemoradiotherapy (CRT)], and indeed, more recently, CRT alone has been used as a curative treatment.[21-23] Previous meta-analyses have demonstrated significant advantages for neoadjuvant treatment regarding local tumour control and disease-free survival;[24,25] however, concern remains regarding the effect on postoperative morbidity and mortality. A meta-analysis sought to clarify the benefits of neoadjuvant and definitive treatment for oesophageal SCC.[26] Morbidity (p = 0.638) and mortality (p = 0.810) rates were not increased by neoadjuvant chemotherapy, and no increase in morbidity was associated with neoadjuvant CRT (p = 0.363). Two RCTs reported increased mortality rates after neodjuvant CRT but the result was not significant. Whilst the R0 resection rates were significantly increased by both neoadjuvant CRT and neoadjuvant chemotherapy compared with surgery alone, a survival benefit was only demonstrated for neoadjuvant

CRT. None of the RCTs reporting outcome after CRT alone demonstrated a significant survival benefit, but treatment-related mortality rates were lower (p = 0.007) than with neoadjuvant treatment followed by surgery or surgery alone.

The JCOG9907 trial previously reported superior progression free and overall survival with neoadjuvant chemotherapy for clinical stage II/III SCC of the thoracic oesophagus compared to adjuvant chemotherapy.[27] Now the safety analysis shows that neoadjuvant chemotherapy is not associated with an increase in postoperative complications.[28]

> **Key Point**
>
> Neoadjuvant chemotherapy for oesophageal SCC results in a significant survival benefit with no increase in morbidity rate. Whilst definitive CRT is associated with lower mortality rates, no demonstrable survival benefit was found over other treatment strategies.

Postoperative Management

Early enteral nutrition (EEN) forms a key part of enhanced recovery programmes after surgery. An RCT randomised 121 patients to either EEN via a feeding jejunostomy or nothing by mouth (NBM) and intravenous fluids following surgery for oesophageal, gastric and pancreatic cancer.[29] Operative morbidity was less common after EEN (32.8%) than control management (50.9%; p = 0.044) due to fewer wound infections (p = 0.017), chest infections (p = 0.036) and anastomotic leaks (p = 0.055). Median length of hospital stay was 16 days after EEN compared with 19 days after control management (p = 0.023). This trial lacked an appropriate control arm (early oral feeding), and the postoperative hospital stay is longer than in most Western centres.

HEPATOPANCREATOBILIARY

Liver

The Pringle manoeuvre[30] is frequently employed to minimise blood loss during transection of hepatic parenchyma. There is interest in whether ischaemic preconditioning (IPC) prior to Pringle manoeuvre can reduce ischaemia-reperfusion injury in the liver remnant. Eighty-four patients were randomised in a trial to either IPC (10 minutes inflow occlusion followed by 10 minutes reperfusion) or no IPC[31] with the primary endpoint being alanine aminotransferase (ALT) level on day 1 postoperatively. The ALT levels on the day after operation were not decreased by IPC, and indeed liver biochemistry tests in the week after operation showed the same pattern in both groups. Intraoperative morbidity and postoperative outcomes were also similar.

> **Key Point**
>
> Ischaemic preconditioning prior to Pringle manoeuvre did not improve either clinical or biochemical outcomes. It remains widely accepted however that intermittent portal clamping reduces ischaemia-reperfusion injury.

Pancreatic

Pancreatic surgery remains a high-risk low-volume specialty and in the UK, it is recommended that patients be treated in specialised pancreatic centres serving a population of 2–4 million.[32] Indeed in a meta-analysis, 9 of 11 studies showed a significant association between higher hospital volume and lower postoperative mortality.[33] Whilst the effect of surgeon volume on postoperative mortality was not significant, previous studies have attributed part of the effect of hospital volume to surgeon volume.[34,35]

Pancreatic fistula formation following distal pancreatectomy represents a major source of postoperative morbidity (13–64%).[36] A multicentre RCT randomly assigned patients to stapler or hand-sewn closure of the pancreatic remnant.[37] The trial found no reduction in postoperative pancreatic fistula and mortality upto postoperative day 7 by stapler resection and closure (stapler 56/177 (32%) versus hand-sewn closure 49/175 (28%); p = 0.56). Of interest, a *post hoc* multivariable analysis did not show any effect of intraoperative and postoperative somatostatin application on pancreatic fistula formation.

> **Key Point**
>
> Stapler closure did not reduce the rate of pancreatic fistula compared with hand-sewn closure for distal pancreatectomy.

Biliary

Between 9% and 19% of patients undergoing laparoscopic cholecystectomy have common bile duct (CBD) stones.[38-40] The options for treatment include open CBD exploration, laparoscopic CBD exploration (LCBDE) or endoscopic sphincterotomy (ES).[41,42] Endoscopic sphincterotomy is often preferred[43-45] since laparoscopic CBD exploration is challenging. Traditionally, endoscopic retrograde cholangiopancreatography (ERCP)/ ES is performed preoperatively; however, there is increasing interest in intraoperative ERCP/ES (IOES). A meta-analysis of four trials comparing preoperative ES with IOES found no significant difference in rate of endoscopic clearance of CBD stones between the groups.[46] Post-ERCP/ES complications such as pancreatitis, bleeding or perforation were lower in the IOES group (3.4% vs 9.3%, p = 0.009). There was no significant difference in laparoscopic cholecystectomy (LC) postoperative morbidity or rate of conversion to open between the groups. Of the two trials that reported length of hospital stay this was shorter in the IOES group (1–5 vs 3–8 days; p < 0.001).

A further trial randomised 226 patients to LC combined with IOES or LC with LCBDE.[47] There was no significant difference in the success rate of CBD clearance between the two interventions (92% for LC-LCBDE vs 97.2% for LC-IOES). Similarly, no differences were found in terms of surgical time and postoperative length of stay. Predictably pancreatitis and bleeding sphincterotomy were significantly more prevalent in the LC-IOES group, whilst bile leakage and retained CBD stones were significantly more prevalent in the LC-LCBDE group.

Intraoperative cholangiography (IOC) is a useful tool for the diagnosis of common bile duct stones and to delineate anatomy. One ninety patients with a history of biliary colic or cholecystitis, and a low predictive risk for choledocholithiasis were randomised to undergo elective LC alone or elective LC with IOC.[48] The incidence of CBD stones was 3%. Whilst four patients in the surgery alone arm were readmitted, three with symptoms and signs suggestive of passage of a stone, none required any intervention. The use of routine cholangiography resulted in three successful LCBDEs. There was one major biliary injury in the surgery alone arm but the study was not powered to assess the impact of routine IOC on the prevention of CBD injury. Whilst this trial demonstrated that IOC was safe and yielded clinically useful information, the operating time was significantly longer and there was no significant difference in the readmission rate at 1 year.

> **Key Point**
>
> Present results do not support the routine use of intraoperative cholangiography in patients with a low predictive risk of CBD stones.

Postoperative pain is a key cause of prolonged stay after LC. Eighty patients were randomised to pre-incisional infiltration and preoperative intraperitoneal instillation of 80 mL of either 0.125% levobupivacaine (experimental group) or normal saline (placebo group).[49] No significant difference was found between the groups. Other modalities to decrease postoperative pain and improve cosmesis after LC include the laparoendoscopic single site (LESS) approach. Of 150 patients randomised to either LESS or conventional LC, better pain profiles and lower analgesic requirements (p < 0.001), and quality of life/body image (p < 0.001) were recorded in the LESS group.[50] Operating times and complications were similar in the two groups.

> **Key Point**
>
> Whilst CL with three or more ports remains the 'gold standard' for cholecystectomy, there is increasing interest in the single-site approach.

COLORECTAL

Colonoscopy/Bowel Imaging

Whilst colonoscopy is the reference standard against which the sensitivity of other colorectal cancer screening tests are compared,[51-53] it does still miss polyps and cancers.[54-56] The narrow band imaging (NBI) technology in conventional video colonoscopes uses special filters to narrow a light source, eliminating red, enhancing structures and rendering vascular structures in black.[57-61] During instrument withdrawal, 482 patients were randomised to either conventional colonoscopy or NBI.[62] No difference was found in the mean number of polyps or adenomas detected. Another study showed more promising results. It evaluated whether enhanced mucosal contrast using pancolonic chromoendoscopy (PCC) allowed higher rates of adenoma detection.[63] A total of 1,008 patients were randomised to either PCC (with 0.4% indigo carmine spraying during continuous extubation) or standard colonoscopy. Pancolonic chromoendoscopy was found to significantly increase the overall detection rate for adenomas (0.95 vs 0.66 per patient p < 0.001), and there was a nonsignificant trend towards increased detection of advanced adenomas (103 vs 81; p = 0.067).

Key to the success of colonoscopy is adequate bowel preparation. A trial examined four different regimes: (1) 4 L polyethylene glycol (PEG); (2) 2 L PEG + 20 mg bisacodyl; (3) 90 mL of sodium phosphate (NaP); or (4) two sachets of a commercially available bowel cleansing solution (PSMC) + 300 mL of magnesium citrate (M).[64] The mean total cleansing score was significantly worse in the NaP group compared with the other groups (p < 0.0001). A short interval between completion of bowel preparation and start of colonoscopy was the most important predictor of bowel cleanliness. In a different trial, 190 patients were randomised to either MiraLAX, 103 or Golytely with the finding that Golytely was more efficacious.[65]

Colorectal Cancer

The use of total mesorectal excision (TME) has led to substantial improvements in survival following surgery for rectal cancer.[66] The TME trial has previously reported the value of short-term radiotherapy in combination with TME, and early results showed a decreased risk of local recurrence for irradiated patients at 2 years (2% vs 8%; p < 0.001).[67] At a follow-up of 10 years, the group now report a cumulative incidence of local recurrence of 5% in the preoperative radiotherapy group compared to 11% in the surgery-alone group (p < 0.0001).[68] Interestingly, this did not translate into an overall survival benefit except in patients with a negative circumferential margin and TNM stage III.

> **Key Point**
>
> Whilst short-term radiotherapy in combination with TME appears to reduce the incidence of local recurrence, this does not translate into an overall survival benefit for all patients.

Colonic stenting can restore luminal patency avoiding the need for emergency surgery in patients with left-sided colorectal cancer presenting with bowel obstruction. A trial randomised patients with acute obstructed left-sided cancer to emergency surgery or colonic stenting as a bridge to surgery.[69] However, in accordance with the advice of the data safety monitoring committee, the study was halted due to increased morbidity within the colonic stenting group. The most common serious adverse events were abscess (three in the colonic stenting group vs four in the emergency surgery group), perforations (six vs none) and anastomotic leakage (five vs one).

The laparoscopic approach is now commonplace in colorectal cancer surgery. An RCT evaluated the cost-effectiveness of bipolar vessel sealer (BVS)

compared with clips and vascular stapler (CVS) in laparoscopic colorectal resection.[70] In multivariable analysis, the cost of disposable instruments for vascular control was independently reduced by randomisation to BVS, type of procedure, female sex and estimated blood loss. The mean cost reduction was $88.2 for left colectomy (p = 0.037), $377.7 (p = 0.005) for total colectomy and $366.9 (p = 0.012) for proctectomy. Conversely, use of the BVS increased the cost of instruments used for vascular control in right colectomy by $92.6 (p = 0.012).

Pelvic Floor Disorders

Pelvic floor disorders encompass a broad range of conditions. A randomised study of patients with faecal incontinence compared injection of nonanimal stabilised hyaluronic acid and dextranomer (NASHA Dx) into the submucosa of the anal sphincter to a sham treatment.[71] A total of 71 patients of 136 assigned to receive NASHA Dx (52%) had a 50% or more reduction in the number of incontinence episodes compared to 22 of 70 patients who received the *sham* treatment (31%; p = 0.0089).

A number of abdominal procedures are available for the treatment of full-thickness rectal prolapse (FTRP). These differ technically as to whether rectopexy is added to mobilisation of the rectum. In a multicentre RCT, patients with FTRP were assigned to either rectopexy or no rectopexy.[72] There was a marked difference in 5-year recurrence rates between study arms (1.5% vs 8.6%; p = 0.003); hence, the study concluded that recurrence rates following no rectopexy are inferior to those following rectopexy for external FTRP.

Anorectal function is often impaired after low anterior resection of the rectum. A trial aimed to assess whether a temporary defunctioning stoma affected anorectal function after patients had been stoma-free for a year.[73] Defunctioning stoma did not affect anorectal function. However, because this study was an analysis of secondary end points of a randomised trial, no pre-study power calculation was performed.

BREAST AND ENDOCRINE

Benign Breast Disease

The harmonic scalpel utilises ultrasonic energy for resecting tissues and providing haemostasis. A total of 31 patients undergoing bilateral breast reduction surgery were evaluated in a matched-pair design, with random (blinded) assignment of one side to the harmonic scalpel, with the other side defaulting to electrocautery.[74] No statistical differences were found in terms of resection/haemostasis time, drainage volume and postoperative pain. Whilst more complications were noted with the use of the harmonic scalpel, this did not reach statistical significance; however, the sample size was small. The authors concluded that whilst the harmonic device may be excellent for other surgical procedures, its high cost suggests that surgeons and institutions can confidently forgo its use in breast reduction surgery.

Breast Cancer

Axillary lymph node dissection (ALND) is the standard of care for patients in whom sentinel lymph node (SLN) biopsy identifies metastases,[75] but it is not without morbidity. However, with increasing knowledge of the complexity of tumour biology, lymph node status now influences rather than dictates the use of chemotherapy.[76-81] To determine the need for ALND, 891 women with clinical T1-T2 invasive breast cancer, no palpable adenopathy, and 1–2 SLNs containing metastases, undergoing lumpectomy and radiation therapy were randomised to either complete ALND (dissection of 10 or more nodes) or no further axillary treatment.[82] At a median follow-up of 6.3 years, OS and DFS were equivalent.

> **Key Point**
>
> Women with a positive SLN and clinical T1-T2 tumours undergoing lumpectomy with radiation therapy followed by systemic therapy do not benefit from the addition of ALND in terms of local control, disease-free survival or overall survival.

Finally, a review of a historical trial commenced in 1982 comprising 200 patients aged 70 or over with operable breast cancer randomised to surgery or tamoxifen with crossover on recurrence found that whilst 50% of deaths from breast cancer occurred within the first 5 years of follow-up, further deaths occurred upto 25 years later.[83] This reiterates the belief that there is never a time after treatment when it can be stated that a patient is cured of breast cancer.

> **Key Points**
>
> 1. Urgent appendicectomy remains the recommended treatment for acute uncomplicated appendicitis.
>
> 2. In patients with BMI 25–35, gastric bypass is more likely to achieve remission of T2DM than sleeve gastrectomy.
>
> 3. Neoadjuvant chemotherapy for oesophageal SCC results in a significant survival benefit with no increase in morbidity rate. Whilst definitive CRT is associated with lower mortality rates, no demonstrable survival benefit was found over other treatment strategies.
>
> 4. Ischaemic preconditioning prior to Pringle manoeuvre did not improve either clinical or biochemical outcomes. It remains widely accepted however that intermittent portal clamping reduces ischaemia-reperfusion injury.

REFERENCES

1. Vons C, Barry C, Maitre S, et al. Amoxicillin plus clavulanic acid versus appendicectomy for treatment of acute uncomplicated appendicitis: an open-label, non-inferiority, randomised controlled trial. Lancet. 2011;377(9777):1573-9.
2. Eriksen R, Bisgaard T, Assaadzadeh S, et al. Randomized clinical trial of fibrin sealant versus titanium tacks for mesh fixation in laparoscopic umbilical hernia repair. Br J Surg. 2011;98(11):1537-45.
3. Paajanen H, Kössi J, Silvasti S, et al. Randomized clinical trial of tissue glue versus absorbable sutures for mesh fixation in local anaesthetic Lichtenstein hernia repair. Br J Surg. 2011;98(9):1245-51.
4. Bittner R, Leibl BJ, Kraft B, et al. One-year results of a prospective, randomised clinical trial comparing four meshes in laparoscopic inguinal hernia repair (TAPP). Hernia. 2011;15(5):503-10.
5. Smietański M, Bury K, Smietańska IA, et al. Five-year results of a randomised controlled multi-centre study comparing heavy-weight knitted versus low-weight, non-woven polypropylene implants in Lichtenstein hernioplasty. Hernia. 2011;15(5):495-501.
6. Demetrashvili Z, Qerqadze V, Kamkamidze G, et al. Comparison of Lichtenstein and laparoscopic transabdominal preperitoneal repair of recurrent inguinal hernias. Int Surg. 2011;96(3):233-8.
7. Bloemen A, van Dooren P, Huizinga BF, et al. Randomized clinical trial comparing polypropylene or polydioxanone for midline abdominal wall closure. Br J Surg. 2011;98(5):633-9.
8. Lee WJ, Chong K, Ser KH, et al. Gastric bypass vs sleeve gastrectomy for type 2 diabetes mellitus: a randomized controlled trial. Arch Surg. 2011;146(2):143-8.
9. Centre for Public Health Excellence at NICE (UK); National Collaborating Centre for Primary Care (UK). Obesity: the prevention, identification, assessment and management of overweight and obesity in adults and children. NICE Clinical Guidelines, No. 43. London: National Institute for Health and Clinical Excellence (UK); 2006.
10. Hunter JG, Trus TL, Branum GD, et al. Laparoscopic Heller myotomy and fundoplication for achalasia. Ann Surg. 1997;225:655-64.
11. Luostarinen M, Isolauri J, Laitinen J, et al. Fate of Nissen fundoplication after 20 years. A clinical, endoscopical and functional analysis. Gut. 1993;34:1015-20.

5. Stapler closure did not reduce the rate of pancreatic fistula compared with hand-sewn closure for distal pancreatectomy.
6. Present results do not support the routine use of intraoperative cholangiography in patients with a low predictive risk of CBD stones.
7. Whilst CL with three or more ports remains the 'gold standard' for cholecystectomy, there is increasing interest in the single-site approach.
8. Whilst short-term radiotherapy in combination with TME appears to reduce the incidence of local recurrence, this does not translate into an overall survival benefit for all patients.
9. Colonic stenting has a higher rate of complications than emergency surgery in acute colonic obstruction.
10. Women with a positive SLN and clinical T1-T2 tumours undergoing lumpectomy with radiation therapy followed by systemic therapy do not benefit from the addition of ALND in terms of local control, disease-free survival or overall survival.

12. Markar SR, Karthikesalingam AP, Wagner OJ, et al. Systematic review and meta-analysis of laparoscopic Nissen fundoplication with or without division of the short gastric vessels. Br J Surg. 2011;98(8):1056-62.

13. Engström C, Jamieson GG, Devitt PG, et al. Meta-analysis of two randomized controlled trials to identify long-term symptoms after division of the short gastric vessels during Nissen fundoplication. Br J Surg. 2011;98(8):1063-7.

14. Ell C, May A, Pech O, et al. Curative endoscopic resection of early esophageal adenocarcinomas (Barrett's cancer). Gastrointest Endosc. 2007;65:3-10.

15. May A, Gossner L, Pech O, et al. Local endoscopic therapy for intraepithelial high-grade neoplasia and early adenocarcinoma in Barrett's oesophagus: acute-phase and intermediate results of a new treatment approach. Eur J Gastroenterol Hepatol. 2002;14:1085-91.

16. Peters FP, Kara MA, Rosmolen WD, et al. Endoscopic treatment of high-grade dysplasia and early stage cancer in Barrett's esophagus. Gastrointest Endosc. 2005;61:506-14.

17. Badreddine RJ, Prasad GA, Wang KK, et al. Prevalence and predictors of recurrent neoplasia after ablation of Barrett's esophagus. Gastrointest Endosc. 2010;71:697-703.

18. Pech O, Behrens A, May A, et al. Long-term results and risk factor analysis for recurrence after curative endoscopic therapy in 349 patients with high-grade intraepithelial neoplasia and mucosal adenocarcinoma in Barrett's oesophagus. Gut. 2008;57:1200-6.

19. Pouw RE, Sharma VK, Bergman JJ, et al. Radiofrequency ablation for total Barrett's eradication: a description of the endoscopic technique, its clinical results and future prospects. Endoscopy. 2008;40:1033-40.

20. van Vilsteren FG, Pouw RE, Seewald S, et al. Stepwise radical endoscopic resection versus radiofrequency ablation for Barrett's oesophagus with high-grade dysplasia or early cancer: a multicentre randomised trial. Gut. 2011;60(6):765-73.

21. Gebski V, Burmeister B, Smithers BM, et al. Survival benefits from neoadjuvant chemoradiotherapy or chemotherapy in oesophageal carcinoma: a meta-analysis. Lancet Oncol. 2007;8:226-34.

22. Bedenne L, Michel P, Bouché O, et al. Chemoradiation followed by surgery compared with chemoradiation alone in squamous cancer of the esophagus: FFCD 9102. J Clin Oncol. 2007;25:1160-8.

23. Stahl M, Stuschke M, Lehmann N, et al. Chemoradiation with and without surgery in patients with locally advanced squamous cell carcinoma of the esophagus. J Clin Oncol. 2005;23:2310-7.

24. Kaklamanos IG, Walker GR, Ferry K, et al. Neoadjuvant treatment for resectable cancer of the esophagus and the gastroesophageal junction: a meta-analysis of randomized clinical trials. Ann Surg Oncol. 2003;10:754-61.

25. Urschel JD, Vasan H. A meta-analysis of randomized controlled trials that compared neoadjuvant chemoradiation and surgery to surgery alone for resectable esophageal cancer. Am J Surg. 2003;185:538-43.

26. Kranzfelder M, Schuster T, Geinitz H, et al. Meta-analysis of neoadjuvant treatment modalities and definitive non-surgical therapy for oesophageal squamous cell cancer. Br J Surg. 2011;98(6):768-83.

27. Igaki H, Ando N, Shinoda M, et al. A randomized trial of postoperative adjuvant chemotherapy with cisplatin and 5-fluorouracil versus neoadjuvant chemotherapy for clinical stage II/III squamous cell carcinoma of the thoracic esophagus (JCOG 9907). J Clin Oncol. 2008; 26(Suppl):Abstract 4510.

28. Hirao M, Ando N, Tsujinaka T, et al. Influence of preoperative chemotherapy for advanced thoracic oesophageal squamous cell carcinoma on perioperative complications. Br J Surg. 2011;98(12):1735-41.

29. Barlow R, Price P, Reid TD, et al. Prospective multicentre randomised controlled trial of early enteral nutrition for patients undergoing major upper gastrointestinal surgical resection. Clin Nutr. 2011;30(5):560-6.

30. Pringle JH. Notes on the arrest of hepatic hemorrhage due to trauma. Ann Surg. 1908;48:541-9.

31. Scatton O, Zalinski S, Jegou D, et al. Randomized clinical trial of ischaemic preconditioning in major liver resection with intermittent Pringle manoeuvre. Br J Surg. 2011;98(9):1236-43.

32. NHS Executive. (2001). Guidance on Commissioning Cancer Services: Improving Outcomes in Upper Gastro-intestinal Cancers. The Manual. [online] Available from http://pro.mountvernoncancernetwork.nhs.uk/assets/Uploads/documents/IOG-Upper-GI-Manual.pdf [Accessed August 31, 2012].

33. Gooiker GA, van Gijn W, Wouters MW, et al. Systematic review and meta-analysis of the volume-outcome relationship in pancreatic surgery. Br J Surg. 2011;98(4):485-94.

34. Birkmeyer JD, Stukel TA, Siewers AE, et al. Surgeon volume and operative mortality in the United States. N Engl J Med. 2003;349:2117-27.

35. Nathan H, Cameron JL, Choti MA, et al. The volume-outcomes effect in hepato-pancreato-biliary surgery: hospital versus surgeon contributions and specificity of the relationship. J Am Coll Surg. 2009;208:528-38.

36. Andren-Sandberg A, Wagner M, Tihanyi T, et al. Technical aspects of left-sided pancreatic resection for cancer. Dig Surg. 1999;16(4):305-12.

37. Diener MK, Seiler CM, Rossion I, et al. Efficacy of stapler versus hand-sewn closure after distal pancreatectomy (DISPACT): a randomised, controlled multicentre trial. Lancet. 2011;377(9776):1514-22.

38. Hainsworth PJ, Rhodes M, Gompertz RH, et al. Imaging of the common bile duct in patients undergoing laparoscopic cholecystectomy. Gut. 1994;35:991-5.

39. Ausch C, Hochwarter G, Taher M, et al. Improving the safety of laparoscopic cholecystectomy: the routine use of preoperative magnetic resonance cholangiography. Surg Endosc. 2005;19:574-80.

40. Yang MH, Chen TH, Wang SE, et al. Biochemical predictors for absence of common bile duct stones in patients undergoing laparoscopic cholecystectomy. Surg Endosc. 2008;22:1620-4.

41. Hong DF, Xin Y, Chen DW. Comparison of laparoscopic cholecystectomy combined with intraoperative endoscopic sphincterotomy and laparoscopic exploration of the common bile duct for cholecystocholedocholithiasis. Surg Endosc. 2006;20:424-7.

42. Martin DJ, Vernon DR, Toouli J. Surgical versus endoscopic treatment of bile duct stones. Cochrane Database Syst Rev. 2006;(2):CD003327.

43. Ludwig K, Kockerling F, Hohenberger W, et al. Surgical therapy in cholecysto-/choledocholithiasis. Results of a Germany-wide questionnaire sent to 859 clinics with 123,090 cases of cholecystectomy. Chirurg. 2001;72(10):1171-8.

44. Spelsberg FW, Nusser F, Huttl TK, et al. Management of cholecysto- and choledocholithiasis—survey and analysis of 16,615 cholecystectomies and common bile duct explorations in Bavaria. Zentralbl Chir. 2009;134:120-6.

45. Bingener J, Schwesinger WH. Management of common bile duct stones in a rural area of the United States: results of a survey. Surg Endosc. 2006;20:577-9.

46. Gurusamy K, Sahay SJ, Burroughs AK, et al. Systematic review and meta-analysis of intraoperative versus preoperative endoscopic sphincterotomy in patients with gallbladder and suspected common bile duct stones. Br J Surg. 2011;98(7):908-16.

47. ElGeidie AA, ElShobary MM, Naeem YM. Laparoscopic exploration versus intraoperative endoscopic sphincterotomy for common bile duct stones: a prospective randomized trial. Dig Surg. 2011;28(5-6):424-31.

48. Khan OA, Balaji S, Branagan G, et al. Randomized clinical trial of routine on-table cholangiography during laparoscopic cholecystectomy. Br J Surg. 2011;98(3):362-7.

49. Hilvering B, Draaisma WA, van der Bilt JD, et al. Randomized clinical trial of combined preincisional infiltration and intraperitoneal instillation of levobupivacaine for postoperative pain after laparoscopic cholecystectomy. Br J Surg. 2011;98(6):784-9.

50. Bucher P, Pugin F, Buchs NC, et al. Randomized clinical trial of laparoendoscopic single-site versus conventional laparoscopic cholecystectomy. Br J Surg. 2011;98(12):1695-702.

51. US Preventive Services Task Force. Screening for colorectal cancer: US Preventive Services Task Force recommendation statement. Ann Intern Med. 2008;149(9):627-37.

52. Whitlock EP, Lin JS, Liles E, et al. Screening for colorectal cancer: an updated systematic review. Evidence Synthesis No. 65, Part 1. AHRQ publication no. 08-05124-EF-1. Rockville, MD: Agency for Healthcare Research and Quality; 2008.

53. Whitlock E, Lin JS, Liles E, et al. Screening for colorectal cancer: a targeted systematic review for the US Preventive Services Task Force. Ann Intern Med. 2008;149(9):638-58.

54. van Rijn JC, Reitsma JB, Stoker J, et al. Polyp miss rate determined by tandem colonoscopy: a systematic review. Am J Gastroenterol. 2006;101(2):343-50.

55. Heresbach D, Barrioz T, Lapalus MG, et al. Miss rate for colorectal neoplastic polyps: a prospective multicenter study of back-to-back video colonoscopies. Endoscopy. 2008;40(4):284-90.

56. Postic G, Lewin D, Bickerstaff C, et al. Colonoscopic miss rates determined by direct comparison of colonoscopy with colon resection specimens. Am J Gastroenterol. 2002;97(12):3182-5.

57. Gono K, Obi T, Yamaguchi M, et al. Appearance of enhanced tissue features in narrow-band endoscopic imaging. J Biomed Opt. 2004;9:568-77.

58. Rastogi A, Bansal A, Wani S, et al. Does narrow band imaging (NBI) colonoscopy increase the detection rate of colon polyps? - a pilot feasibility study. Gastrointest Endosc. 2007;65(5):AB259-AB259.

59. Sano Y, Kobayashi M, Hamamoto Y. New diagnostic method based on color imaging using narrow-band imaging (NBI) system for gastrointestinal tract. Gastrointest Endosc. 2001;53:AB125.

60. Machida H, Sano Y, Hamamoto Y, et al. Narrow-band imaging for differential diagnosis of colorectal mucosal lesions: a pilot study. Endoscopy. 2004;36:1094-8.

61. Sano Y, Tajiri H, Shigeaki A. Optical/digital chromoendoscopy during colonoscopy using narrow-band imaging system. Dig Endosc. 2005;17(Suppl 1):S43-S48.

62. Sabbagh LC, Reveiz L, Aponte D, et al. Narrow-band imaging does not improve detection of colorectal polyps when compared to conventional colonoscopy: a randomized controlled trial and meta-analysis of published studies. BMC Gastroenterol. 2011;11:100.

63. Pohl J, Schneider A, Vogell H, et al. Pancolonic chromoendoscopy with indigo carmine versus standard colonoscopy for detection of neoplastic lesions: a randomised two-centre trial. Gut. 2011;60(4):485-90.

64. Kao D, Lalor E, Sandha G, et al. A randomized controlled trial of four precolonoscopy bowel cleansing regimens. Can J Gastroenterol. 2011;25(12):657-62.

65. Enestvedt BK, Fennerty MB, Eisen GM. Randomised clinical trial: MiraLAX vs Golytely - a controlled study of efficacy and patient tolerability in bowel preparation for colonoscopy. Aliment Pharmacol Ther. 2011;33(1):33-40.

66. MacFarlane JK, Ryall RD, Heald RJ. Mesorectal excision for rectal cancer. Lancet. 1993;341(8843):457-60.

67. Kapiteijn E, Marijnen CA, Nagtegaal ID, et al. Preoperative radiotherapy combined with total mesorectal excision for resectable rectal cancer. N Engl J Med. 2001;345(9):638-46.

68. van Gijn W, Marijnen CA, Nagtegaal ID, et al. Preoperative radiotherapy combined with total mesorectal excision for resectable rectal cancer: 12-year follow-up of the multicentre, randomised controlled TME trial. Lancet Oncol. 2011;12(6):575-82.

69. van Hooft JE, Bemelman WA, Oldenburg B, et al. Colonic stenting versus emergency surgery for acute left-sided malignant colonic obstruction: a multicentre randomised trial. Lancet Oncol. 2011;12(4):344-52.

70. Adamina M, Champagne BJ, Hoffman L, et al. Randomized clinical trial comparing the cost and effectiveness of bipolar vessel sealers versus clips and vascular staplers for laparoscopic colorectal resection. Br J Surg. 2011;98(12):1703-12.

71. Graf W, Mellgren A, Matzel KE, et al. Efficacy of dextranomer in stabilised hyaluronic acid for treatment of faecal incontinence: a randomised, sham-controlled trial. Lancet. 2011;377(9770):997-1003.

72. Karas JR, Uranues S, Altomare DF, et al. No rectopexy versus rectopexy following rectal mobilization for full-thickness rectal prolapse: a randomized controlled trial. Dis Colon Rectum. 2011;54(1):29-34.

73. Lindgren R, Hallböök O, Rutegård J, et al. Does a defunctioning stoma affect anorectal function after low rectal resection? Results of a randomized multicenter trial. Dis Colon Rectum. 2011;54(6):747-52.

74. Burdette TE, Kerrigan CL, Homa K. Harmonic scalpel versus electrocautery in breast reduction surgery: a randomized controlled trial. Plast Reconstr Surg. 2011;128(4):243e-249e.

75. Lyman GH, Giuliano AE, Somerfield MR, et al. American Society of Clinical Oncology guideline recommendations for sentinel lymph node biopsy in early-stage breast cancer. J Clin Oncol. 2005;23(30):7703-20.

76. Abrams JS. Adjuvant therapy for breast cancer—results from the USA consensus conference. Breast Cancer. 2001;8(4):298-304.

77. Goldhirsch A, Glick JH, Gelber RD, et al. Meeting highlights: International Consensus Panel on the Treatment of Primary Breast Cancer. J Natl Cancer Inst. 1998;90(21):1601-8.

78. Sørlie T, Perou CM, Tibshirani R, et al. Gene expression patterns of breast carcinomas distinguish tumor subclasses with clinical implications. Proc Natl Acad Sci USA. 2001;98(19):10869-74.

79. van de Vijver MJ, He YD, van't Veer LJ, et al. A gene-expression signature as a predictor of survival in breast cancer. N Engl J Med. 2002;347(25):1999-2009.

80. Albain KS, Barlow WE, Shak S, et al. Prognostic and predictive value of the 21-gene recurrence score assay in postmenopausal women with node-positive, oestrogen-receptor-positive breast cancer on chemotherapy: a retrospective analysis of a randomised trial. Lancet Oncol. 2010;11(1):55-65.

81. Paik S, Tang G, Shak S, et al. Gene expression and benefit of chemotherapy in women with node-negative, estrogen receptor-positive breast cancer. J Clin Oncol. 2006;24(23):3726-34.
82. Giuliano AE, Hunt KK, Ballman KV, et al. Axillary dissection vs no axillary dissection in women with invasive breast cancer and sentinel node metastasis: a randomized clinical trial. JAMA. 2011;305(6):569-75.
83. Gnant M, Mlineritsch B, Stoeger H, et al. Adjuvant endocrine therapy plus zoledronic acid in premenopausal women with early-stage breast cancer: 62-month follow-up from the ABCSG-12 randomised trial. Lancet Oncol. 2011;12(7):631-41.

Index

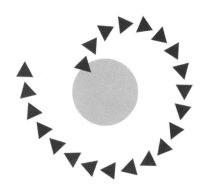

Page numbers followed by *f* refer to figure and *t* refer to table